EAT SO

SMART WAYS TO STAY HEALTHY

Nutritional Food Guide for Vegetarians for A Disease Free Healthy Life

(Full Version)

LA FONCEUR

Copyright © 2019 La Fonceur

All rights reserved.

This book has been published with all efforts taken to make the material error-free. The information on this book is not intended or implied to be a substitute for diagnosis, prognosis, treatment, prescription, and/or dietary advice from a licensed health professional. Author doesn't assume and hereby disclaim any liability to any party for any loss, damage, or disruption caused by errors or omissions, whether such errors or omissions result from negligence, accident, or any other cause.

While every effort has been made to avoid any mistake or omission, this publication is being sold on the condition and understanding that neither the author nor the publishers or printers would be liable in any manner to any person by reason of any mistake or omission in this publication or for any action taken or omitted to be taken or advice rendered or accepted on the basis of this work.

CONTENTS

INTRODUCTION	7
CHAPTER 1	9
PREVENTION IS ACTUALLY BETTER THAN CURE	
CHAPTER 2	13
10 FIBER RICH FOODS FOR BETTER DIGESTION	
CHAPTER 3	24
10 BEST FOODS FOR BETTER SKIN	
CHAPTER 4	35
10 REASONS WHY FAT IS NOT THE ENEMY. THE TRUTH ABOUT FATS!	
CHAPTER 5	47
10 SMART WAYS TO LOSE WEIGHT WITHOUT DIETING	
CHAPTER 6	56
10 REASONS WHY ALCOHOL IS A BIG NO NO!!!	
CHAPTER 7	64
10 REASONS YOU SHOULD START EATING ALMONDS EVERY DAY	
CHAPTER 8	73
10 SMART WAYS TO INCORPORATE PUMPKIN INTO YOUR DIET	
CHAPTER 9	81
RECIPES	

Coconut Burfi Sweet and Healthy	*83*
Spaghetti in Creamy Pumpkin Sauce	*92*
Pumpkin Halwa	*95*
Pumpkin Masala Thepla	*97*
NOTE FROM LA FONCEUR	101
ABOUT THE AUTHOR	102
ALL BOOKS BY LA FONCEUR	103
CONNECT WITH LA FONCEUR	104

INTRODUCTION

Common health problems like indigestion, skin problems, nutritional deficiency, etc., are distressing. They do not interfere much in our day but at the same time do not allow us to live the day with complete satisfaction. We expect these health problems to go away with time, and if they don't, we accept them as part of our life. We tend to think that maybe my skin is naturally sensitive or my digestion is naturally weak, so I am having these problems. The truth is that you don't have to live with these problems. These everyday health problems are the result of an imbalance in the body. Sometimes, this can result from hormonal changes or stress that go away on their own when the stress period ends. But if these problems persist or you have these problems regularly, it means that now you need to make some changes in your diet. Besides stress, these everyday problems are mainly caused by an unbalanced diet or a lack of important nutrients in your diet. By eating the right foods, you can promote the health of your skin and hair, strengthen your digestive system, prevent weight fluctuations, get rid of nutrient deficiencies, and improve your overall health.

Eat So What! Smart Ways to Stay Healthy explains the nutritional value of foods, gives direction on what to eat and gives smart tricks and tips to make life healthier. This book explains how essential nutrients can relieve your everyday health problems and how a balanced diet can promote overall health. It also explains how you can eat everything provided you follow some simple rules.

With **Eat So What! Smart Ways to Stay Healthy**, lose weight without dieting, strengthen digestion, promote skin health, overcome nutritional deficiencies, learn why alcohol is a big no-no, and why fat is not the enemy.

You will also find some healthy and delicious recipes to include in your diet. Now eat healthy without compromising on the taste.

CHAPTER 1

PREVENTION IS ACTUALLY BETTER THAN CURE

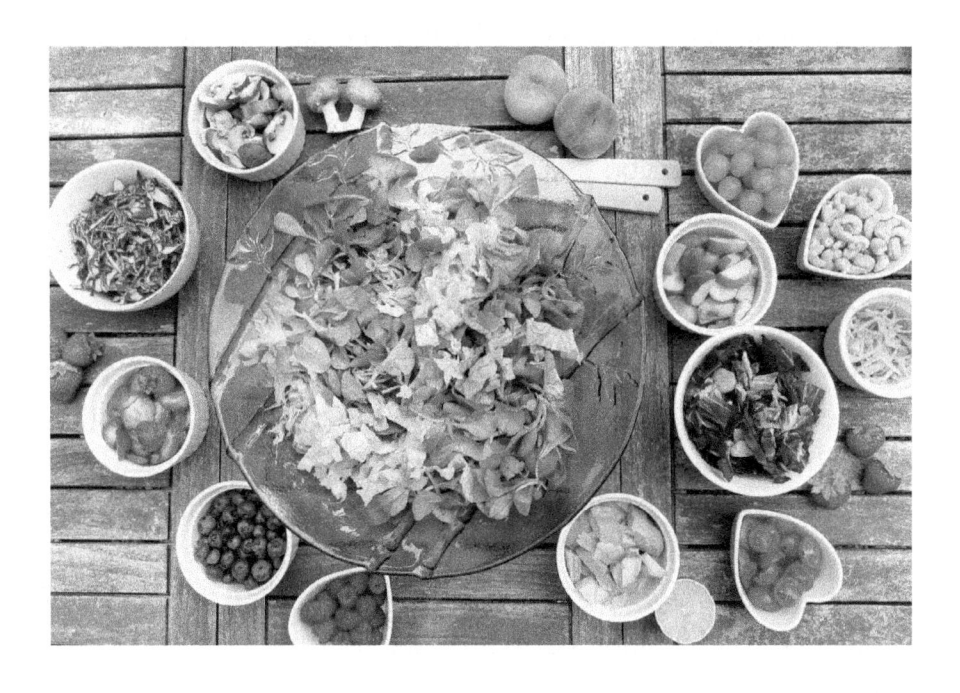

We all know *Prevention is Better Than Cure* but how many of us apply it in our life? The percentage is very low. Usually, when we see someone having a consequence of their bad habits, we tend to assume that this can only happen to others. We tend to think that harmful consequences only happen to others. Somewhere we believe that we are different, it certainly won't happen to me. But the truth is that if you behave irresponsibly towards your health today, sooner or later, you will have to bear the consequences; there is no escape. It may sound harsh, but this is the fact.

The simple rule is that whatever you give to your body, in response, your body will give back the same to you. So, if you are giving junk and health deteriorating elements to your body, you should not expect a healthy life in return. Sometimes our body doesn't immediately alarm for junk and bad habits, and everything seems very normal, but over time, it accumulates, and then it gives you life-threatening diseases. After all, your body needs good care, good food, good lifestyle, and when it is not available to the body, its function gets affected, and over time it loses its functionality.

Many people view their health problems as if God gave them these problems. They don't even consider analyzing whether they have done something wrong that has caused them this particular health problem. I believe that prevention is better than cure. You have to analyze why you are having a specific health problem, what is the root cause, whether it is because of your poor eating habits or poor lifestyle choices? What really went wrong?

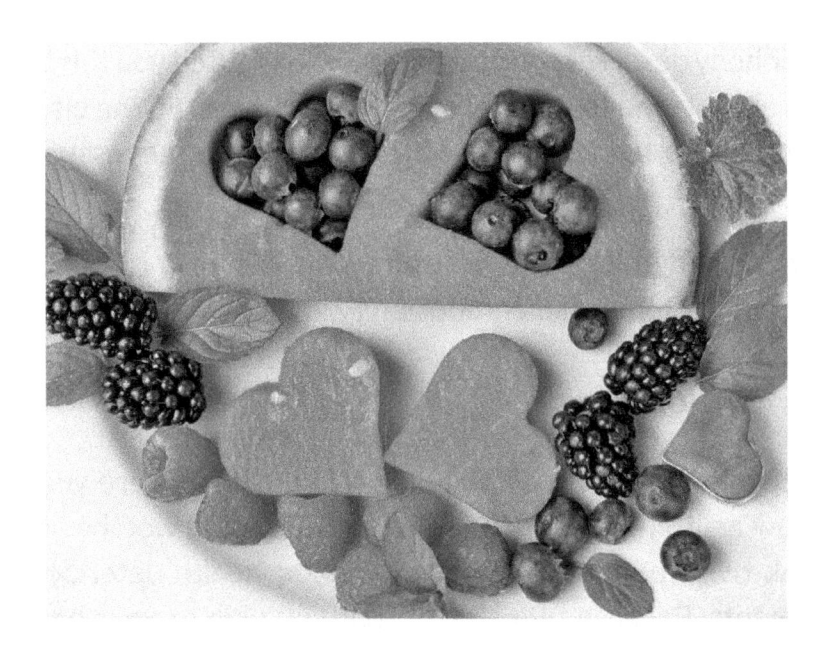

We know that stress causes health problems. What if I ask you to think the opposite? What if I tell you that if you have any health problem, you will be under stress because of that. If you're not feeling healthy, how will you focus on other important aspects of your life? Wouldn't you miss big opportunities in your life because of your health problems?

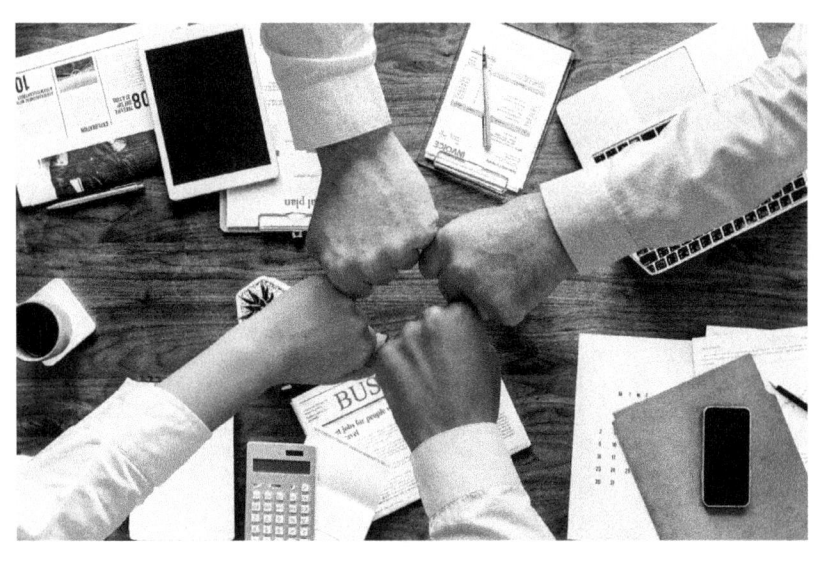

Your body deserves the best care. God has gifted you this body, you are the one to take care of your body, everything else will come and go, but your body will be with you for the rest of your life.

If there is anything you are most responsible for, it is your body. If you don't fulfill your responsibility, then who else will?

Conclusion

Keep in mind that your body is not a dustbin where you can throw anything. This is the temple; You should worship it and think twice before giving it any junk or health deteriorating elements. Because ultimately, what you give to your body, it will give back the same to you.

CHAPTER 2

10 FIBER RICH FOODS FOR BETTER DIGESTION

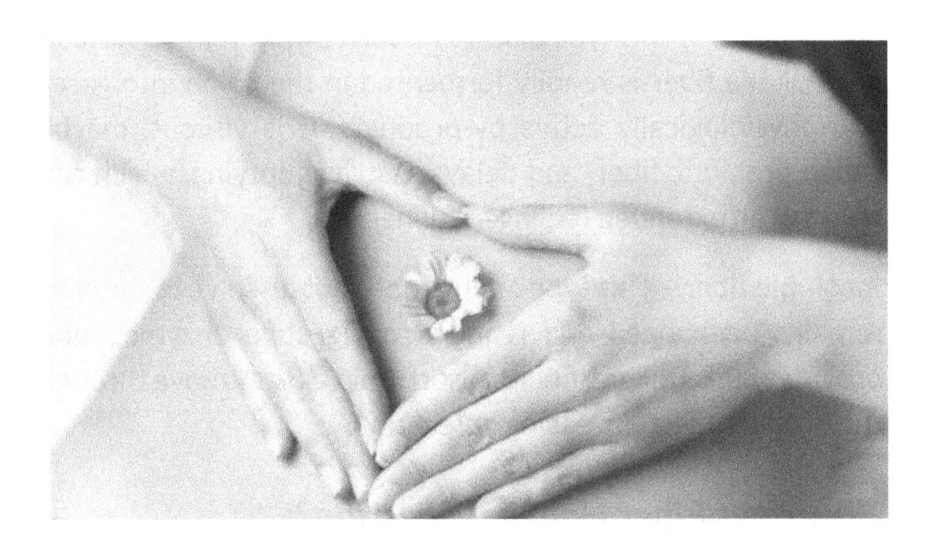

You should eat more fiber. You've probably heard it before. But why is fiber good for your health? Do you know that? Let's dig deeper into it.

What is Dietary Fiber?

Dietary fiber is plant-derived food that digestive enzymes cannot completely break down. It remains unchanged and passes relatively intact through your stomach, small intestine, and colon and out of your body.

Types of Fiber

Soluble fiber – This type of fiber dissolves in water and forms a gel. Soluble fiber is readily fermented in the colon into gases and physiologically active by-products. It is viscous, maybe called prebiotic fiber, and delays gastric emptying, which can result in an extended feeling of fullness.

Insoluble fiber – This type of fiber does not dissolve in water. It remains unchanged and is inert to digestive enzymes, and provides bulk. Bulking fibers absorb fluid as they move through the digestive system, easing defecation.

How does Fiber Help in Digestion?

Fiber plays significant role in keeping your digestive system healthy. The colon cells use fiber to keep them healthy. Soluble fiber dissolves in water, forms a gel, and attaches to cholesterol particles to takes them out of the body, reducing the overall cholesterol levels and the heart disease risk. Insoluble fiber helps to keep the digestive tract flowing by keeping your bowel movements soft and regular.

Below are the 10 fiber-rich foods for your better digestion:

1. Chia Seeds

Chia seeds are tiny black seeds that form a gel when they come in contact with water. They are highly nutritious, containing high amounts of magnesium, phosphorus, and calcium. Chia seeds are very high in fiber.

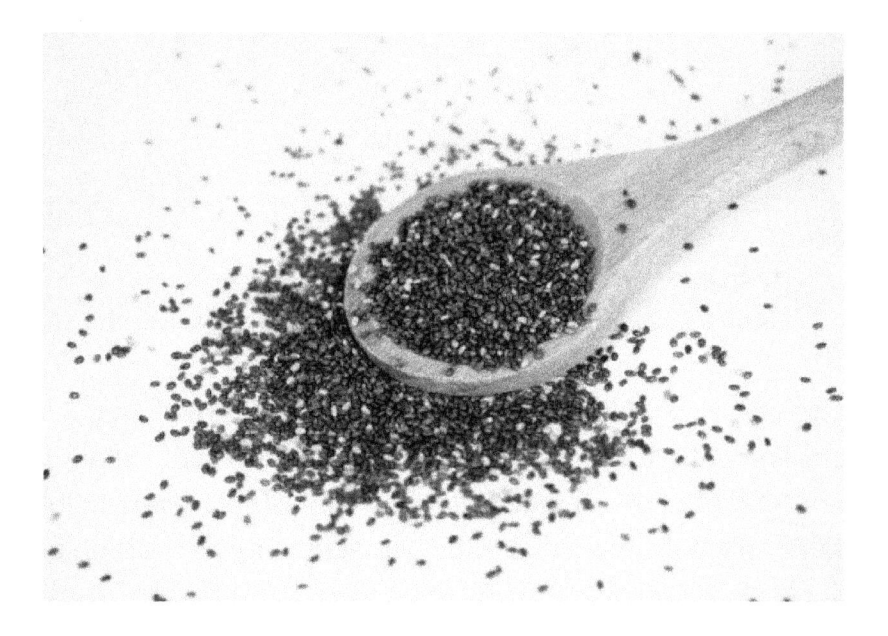

The fiber in chia seeds absorbs a good amount of water and expands in the stomach, keeping you feeling fuller for longer. Chia seeds are rich in fiber, protein, and minerals and perfect for lowering cholesterol levels, boosting bowel movement, and reducing inflammation in the body. Soak chia seeds overnight and eat them for breakfast by adding them to your favorite smoothie to get your daily recommended intake of fiber.

2. Oats

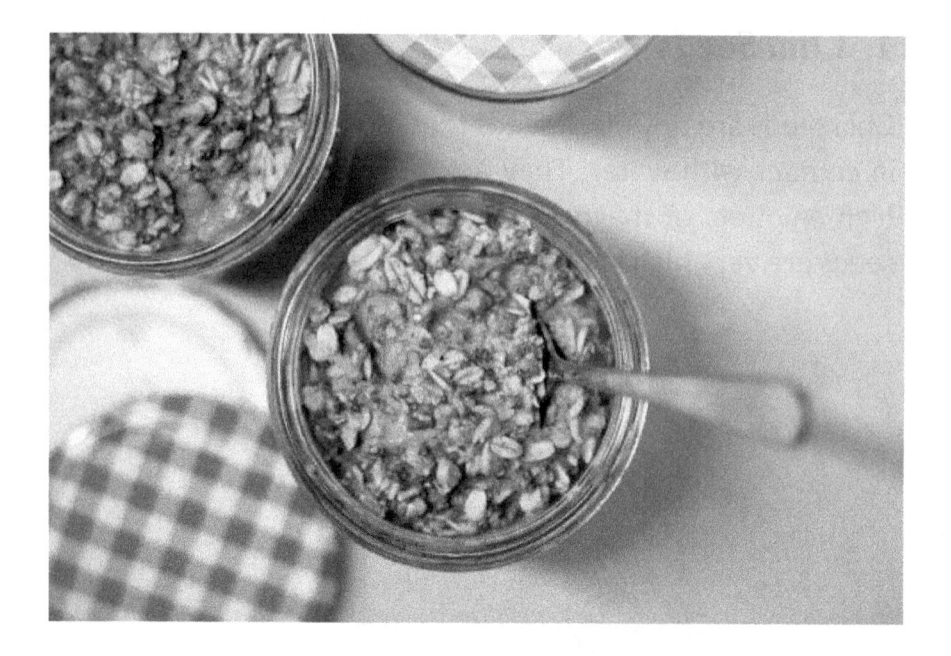

Oats are rich in vitamins, minerals, and antioxidants. They contain beta-glucan, a powerful soluble fiber that has beneficial effects on blood sugar and cholesterol levels. Soluble fiber from oatmeal binds with bile acids in your gut, helping excess cholesterol go out through waste, ultimately lowering your cholesterol levels. As soluble fiber goes through your digestive system, they absorb water and turns into a gel that slows digestion and you feel fuller for a longer period of time. Oats increase the growth of good bacteria in the digestive tract.

3. Chickpeas

Chickpea is a type of legume which is loaded with nutrients, including protein and minerals. They are rich in prebiotic fibers, which act as food for healthy bacteria in your digestive system.

This can lead to a reduced risk of some digestive conditions, such as irritable bowel syndrome and colon cancer. The protein and fiber of chickpeas work synergistically to slow digestion, which helps promote fullness. Chickpeas contain soluble fiber; it blends with water and forms a gel-like substance in the digestive tract.

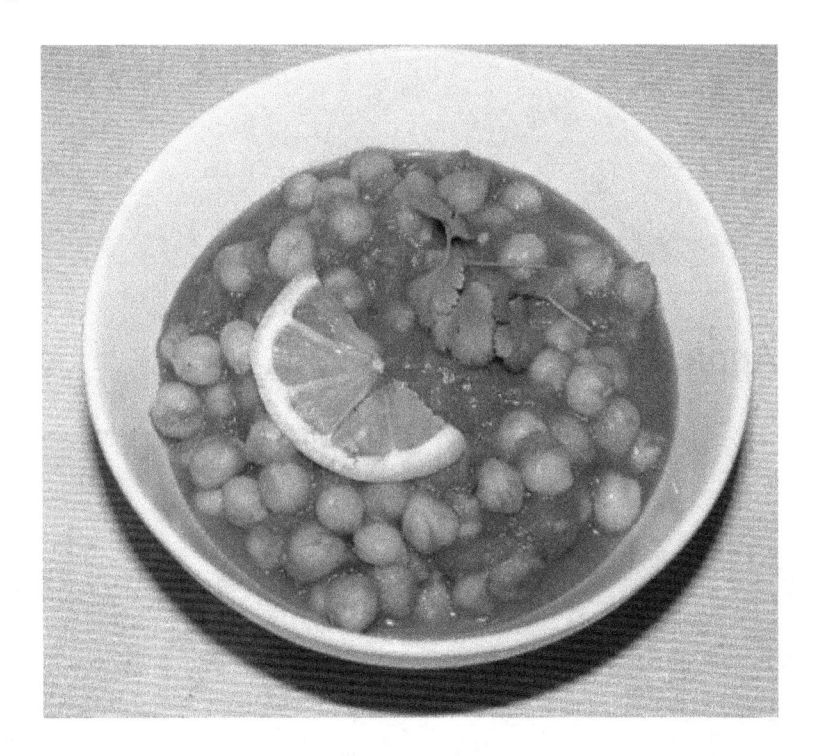

4. Lentils

Lentils are very high in protein and loaded with many important nutrients. Lentils contain both insoluble and soluble fiber. That means they promote weight loss by making you full by expanding in the stomach and absorbing water. Additionally, their fiber carries waste, excess fat, and toxins out of the body and can improve heart health, digestive, immune, and metabolic function.

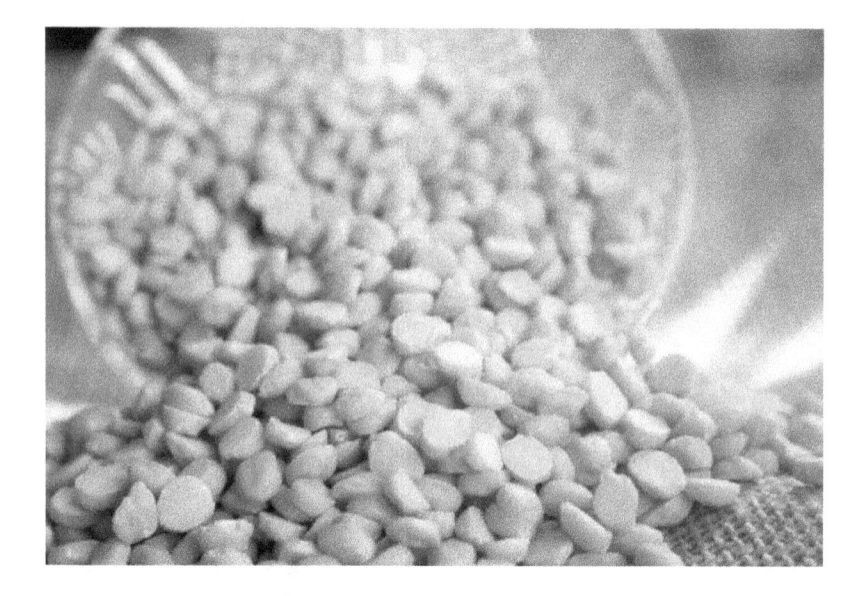

5. Apples

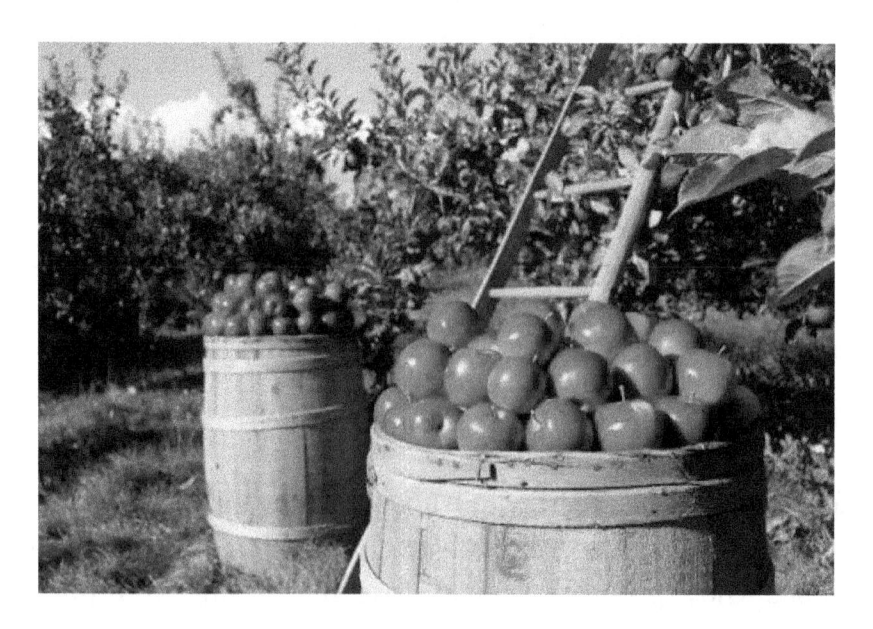

Apples are relatively high in fiber and among the tastiest and most satisfying fruits that you can eat. Apples contain the fiber pectin, which improves digestion as it is soluble in nature and binds to cholesterol and toxins in the body and eliminates them from the body. Due to the high fiber content, an apple makes you feel full; Eating an apple half an hour before a meal results in eating fewer calories in the meal.

6. Sweet Potatoes

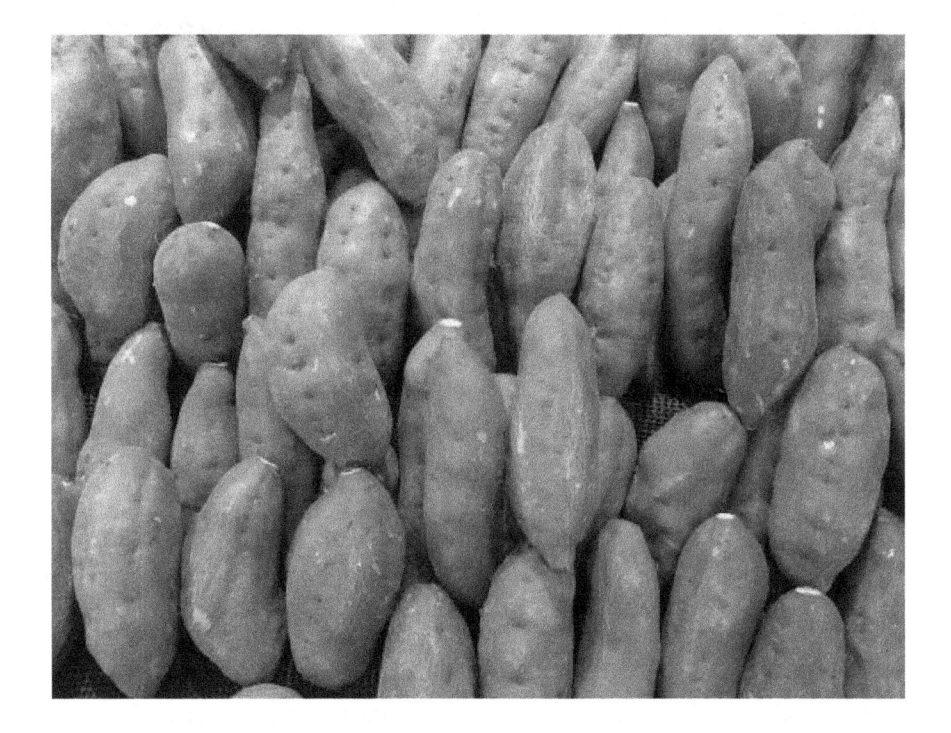

Sweet potatoes are super healthy and have a delicious sweet flavor. They are very high in beta-carotene, B vitamins, and various minerals. Eat sweet potatoes with their skin on. With the skin on, their fiber content gets better. The starchy texture of sweet potatoes contains fiber, which aids digestion. Sweet potatoes are soothing to the stomach and intestines, so they are easily digested and prevent constipation.

7. Kidney Beans

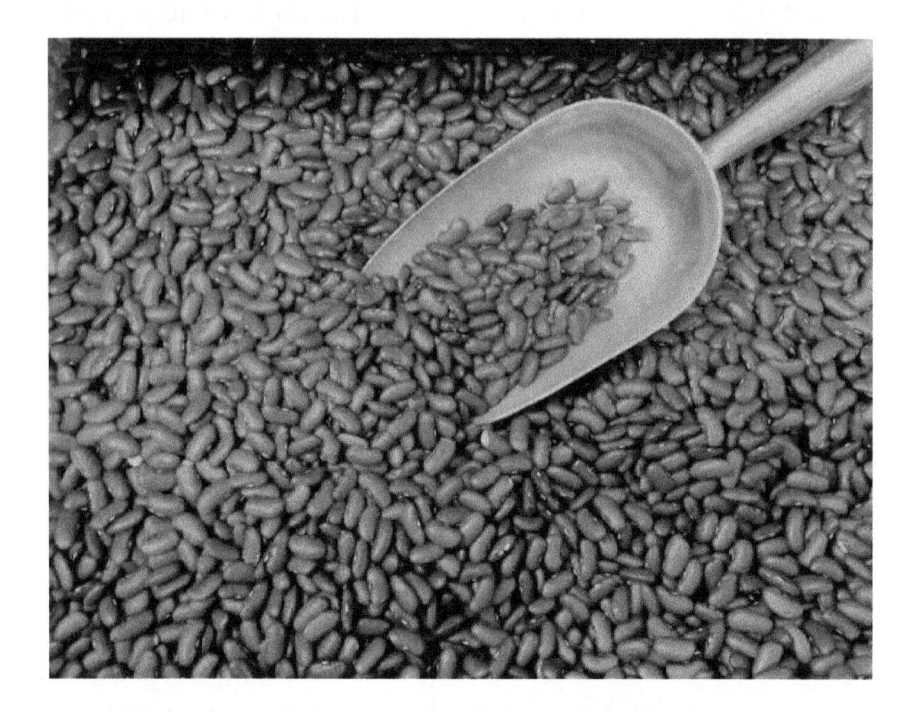

Kidney beans are good for digestion. Kidney beans have both soluble and insoluble fiber, which keeps your digestive system running smoothly. Soluble fiber slows down digestion, which gives you that full feeling, and insoluble fiber helps prevent constipation. But you have to ensure that you do not overindulge to prevent the problems like gas and flatulence.

8. Brussels Sprouts

Brussels sprouts are a type of cruciferous vegetable that resembles mini cabbages. They are high in vitamin K, folate, potassium, and potent cancer-fighting antioxidants as well as dietary fiber. Eating Brussels sprouts and other good sources of fiber like fruits, vegetables, and whole grains can easily help meet your daily recommended fiber requirements.

Brussels sprouts are rich in glucosinates, which can protect the mucosal lining of the GI tract and reduce the risk of digestive disorders.

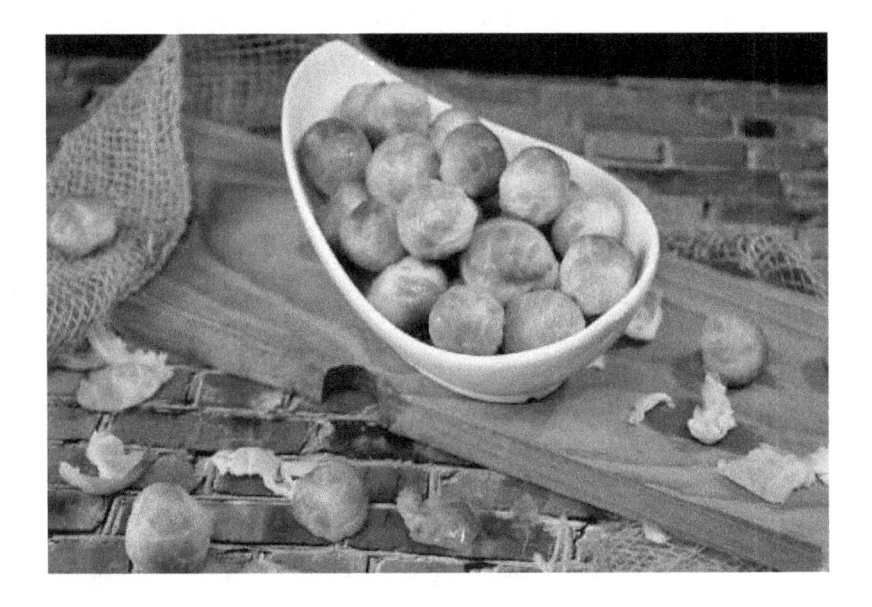

9. Carrots

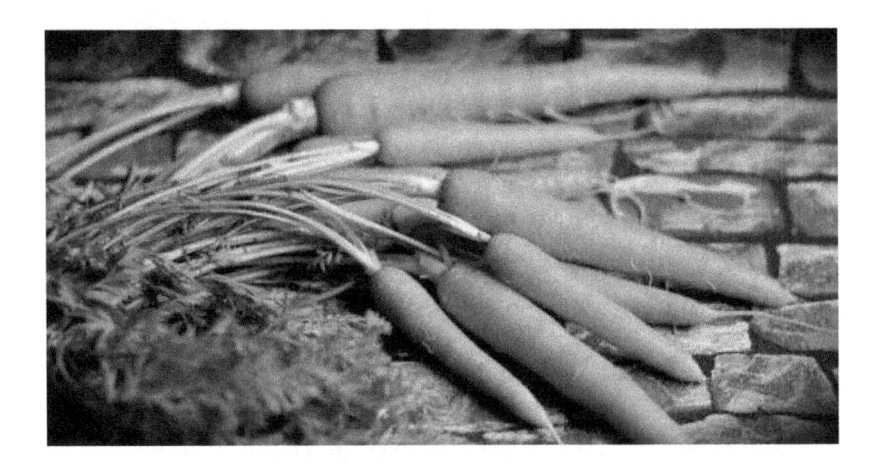

Carrots are high in vitamin K, magnesium, and beta-carotene, an antioxidant that gets turned into vitamin A in the body. Not only for the eyes, but carrots are also good for digestion. They are high in fiber and antioxidants and can help you maintain good digestive health. The soluble fiber in carrots can be beneficial for your digestive system in many ways. This fiber is essential to regulating your digestion and also keep your cholesterol levels healthy.

10. Avocado

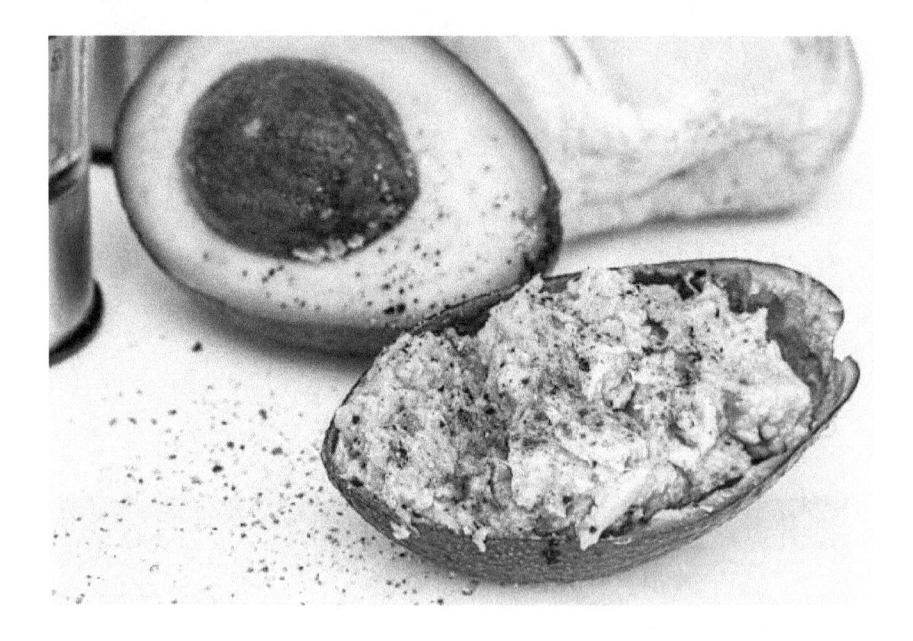

Avocado is great source of fiber. It is super rich in fiber and healthy monounsaturated fats, and essential nutrients, such as potassium, which help promote healthy digestive function. In addition, it helps in the conversion of beta-carotene into vitamin A and aid in the digestion process by maintaining the mucosal lining in the gastrointestinal tract. It's also a low-fructose food, so it's less likely to cause gas. The fiber in avocado can help prevent constipation, maintain a healthy digestive tract, and lower colon cancer risk.

Conclusion

Good digestion is key for a good life. By keeping your digestive system healthy, you can keep many diseases at bay. Fiber-rich foods play an important role in digestion by helping food move through your system more easily or quickly. If you're seeking relief for your digestive woes, consider adding fiber-rich foods to your diet. After all, prevention is better than cure.

CHAPTER 3

10 BEST FOODS FOR BETTER SKIN

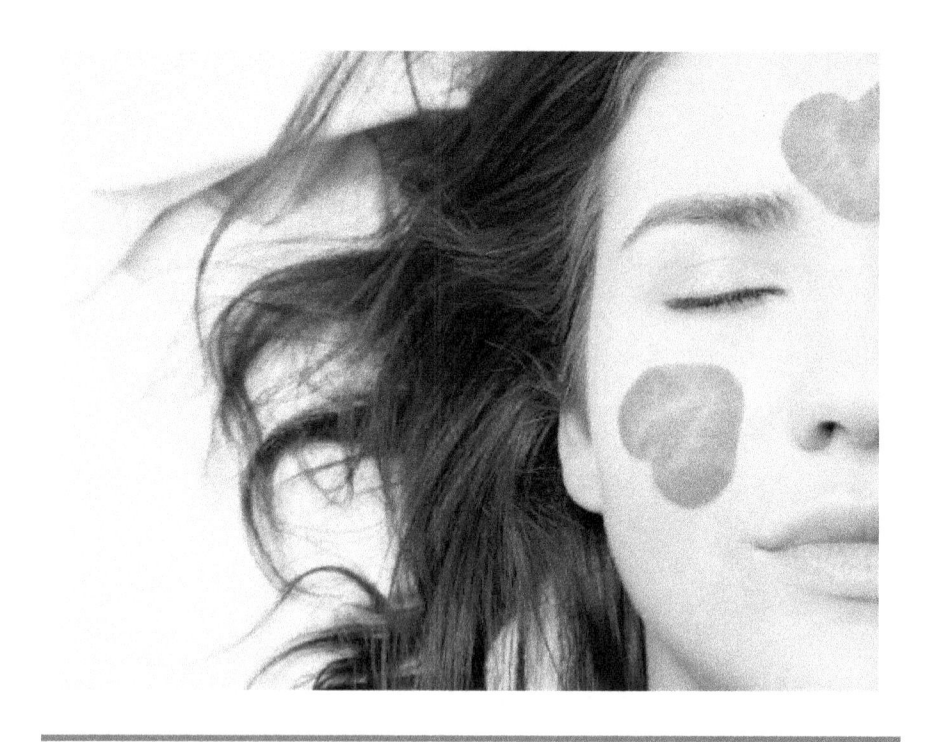

Our life seems to be speeding up and becoming less empathic and increasingly stressful, which puts extra stress on our skin health. Our dependence on processed food is increasing day by day. Processed, refined, and manufactured foods and snacks fuel inflammation on the skin. Skin inflammation can cause redness, acne, and wrinkles.

But nature has the solution to all the problems. We are blessed with some magic foods that protects skin cells from the sun's rays, keep skin hydrated, and limit skin damage from harmful molecules known as free radicals and build strong cell walls for smooth and firm skin.

Below are the 10 best foods for better and healthier skin:

1. Almonds

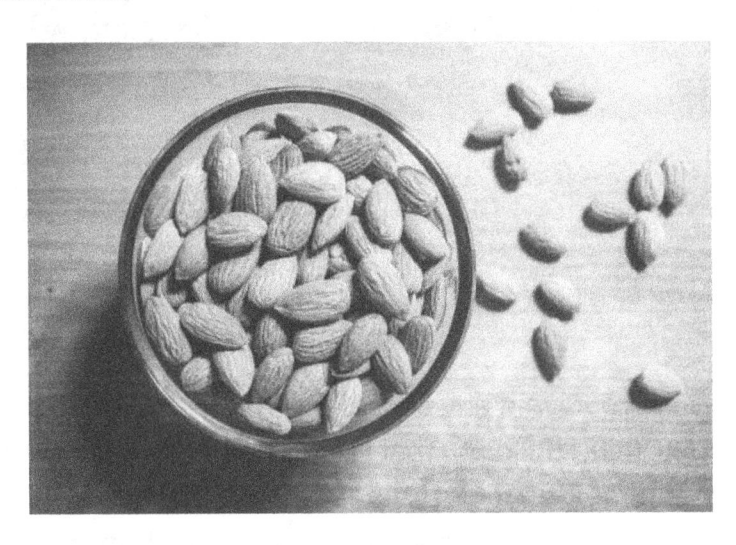

Almonds are a good source of vitamin E and antioxidants. These powerful antioxidants fight free radicals and reduce inflammation, making your skin healthier and younger. People with dermatitis should eat almonds daily. Antioxidants in almonds can fight the damage produced by UV rays, pollution, and a poor diet on the skin. Almonds fight against aging, malnourished skin and prevent skin cancer.

2. Dark Chocolate

Chocolate is derived from cocoa beans, which are rich in flavanols, a potent antioxidant that protects the skin from UV damage, prevents dark spots, premature aging, rashes, and skin cancer. Flavanols boost blood circulation for a healthy glow.

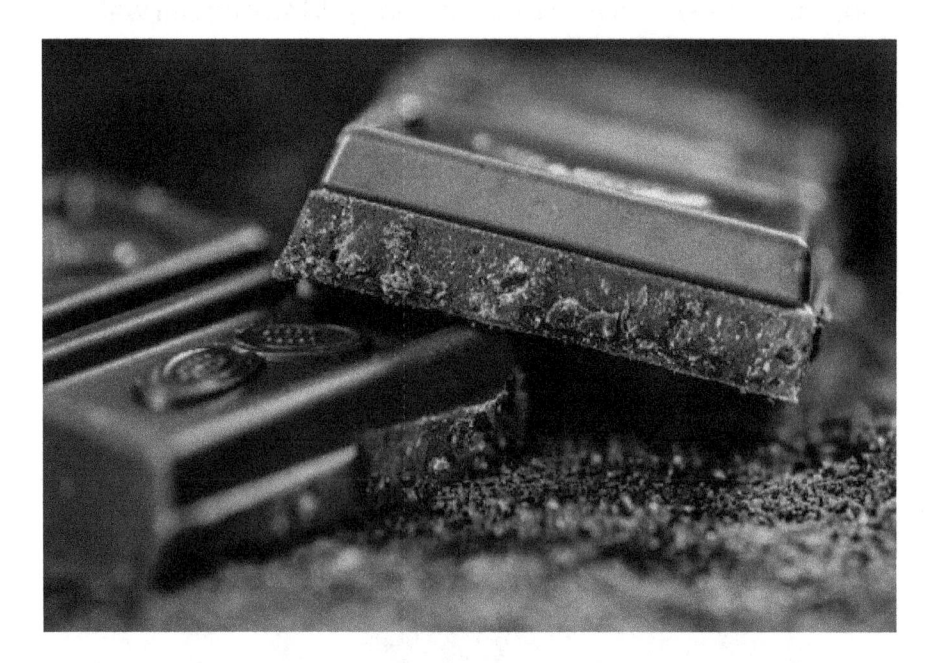

Make sure you avoid any chocolate with less than 70 percent cocoa, like milk chocolate that contain loads of sugar and dairy, which can be terrible for your skin. Go for high cocoa concentrations for the highest concentration of antioxidants to hydrate your skin and improve circulation, leading to healthier, younger-looking skin.

3. Peppers

Yellow and green peppers are an excellent source of beta-carotene, an antioxidant that your body converts into vitamin A.

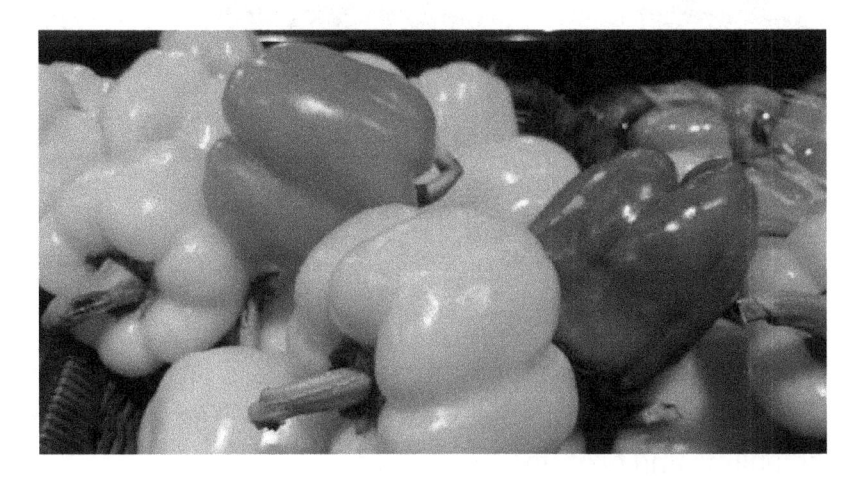

Bell peppers are also one of the best vitamin C sources necessary for creating the protein collagen, which keeps skin firm and strong. Carotenoids decrease sun sensitivity, diminishing the appearance of fine lines around the eyes.

4. Walnuts

Walnuts have both omega-3 and omega-6 fats more than any other nuts. These fatty acids are essential, and your body cannot make them on its own.

Omega-3 fatty acids may improve psoriasis condition or eczema by reducing the inflammatory compounds in the body.

Walnuts contain zinc, which is necessary for wound healing and combatting both bacteria and inflammation.

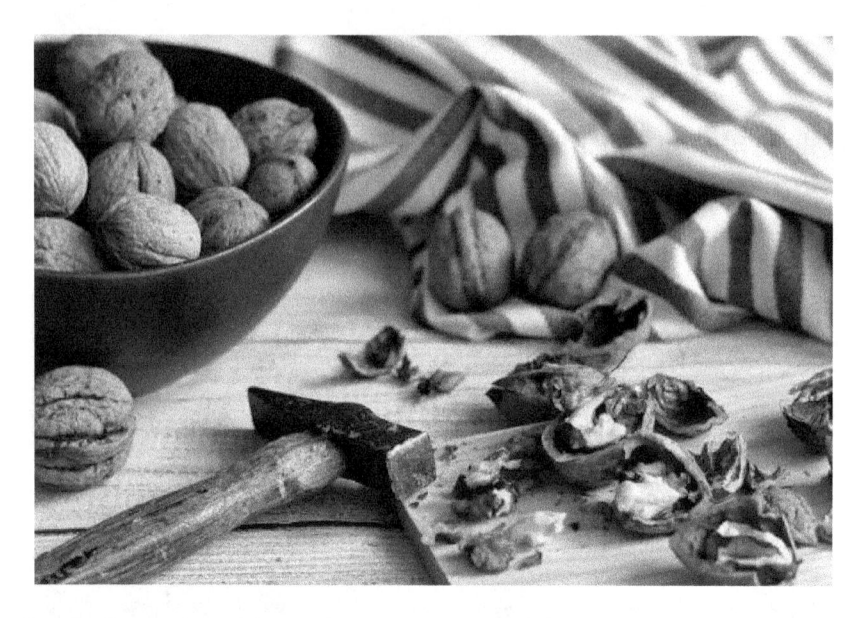

Zinc helps your skin to function properly as a barrier. Walnuts also provide small amounts of antioxidants, vitamin C, vitamin E, selenium, and protein.

5. Tomatoes

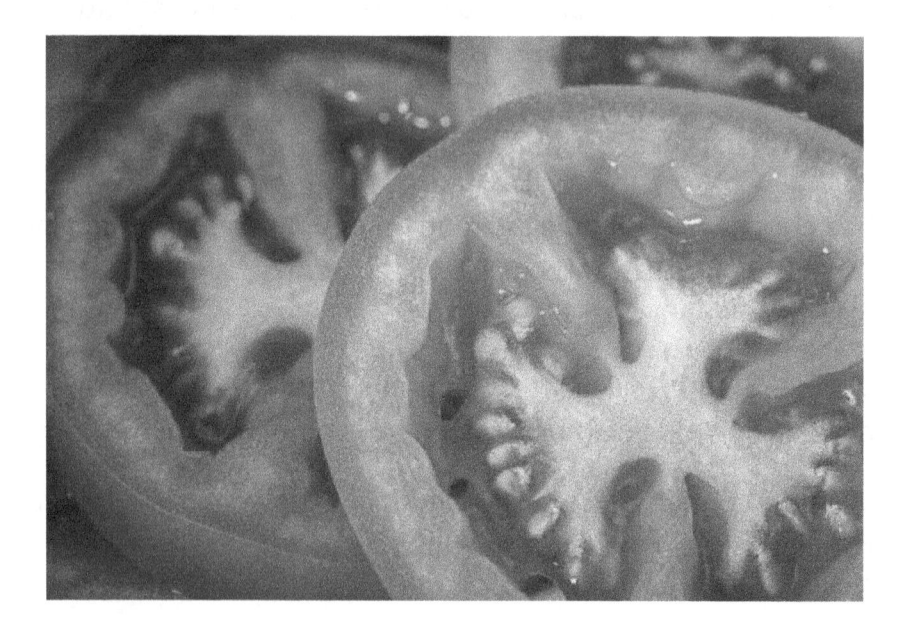

Lycopene is responsible for the bright red color of tomatoes. It is a carotenoid pigment and phytochemical, a potent antioxidant that protects the skin from UV damage. It may also help prevent wrinkling.

Tomatoes are also a great vitamin C source. Fat increases the absorption of carotenoids. Consider pairing tomatoes with a source of fat, like olive oil. Add tomato paste in your face pack paste for instantly glowing skin.

Read 10 Nutrient Combinations You Should Eat for Maximum Health Benefits in the book Eat to Prevent and Control Disease.

6. Green Tea

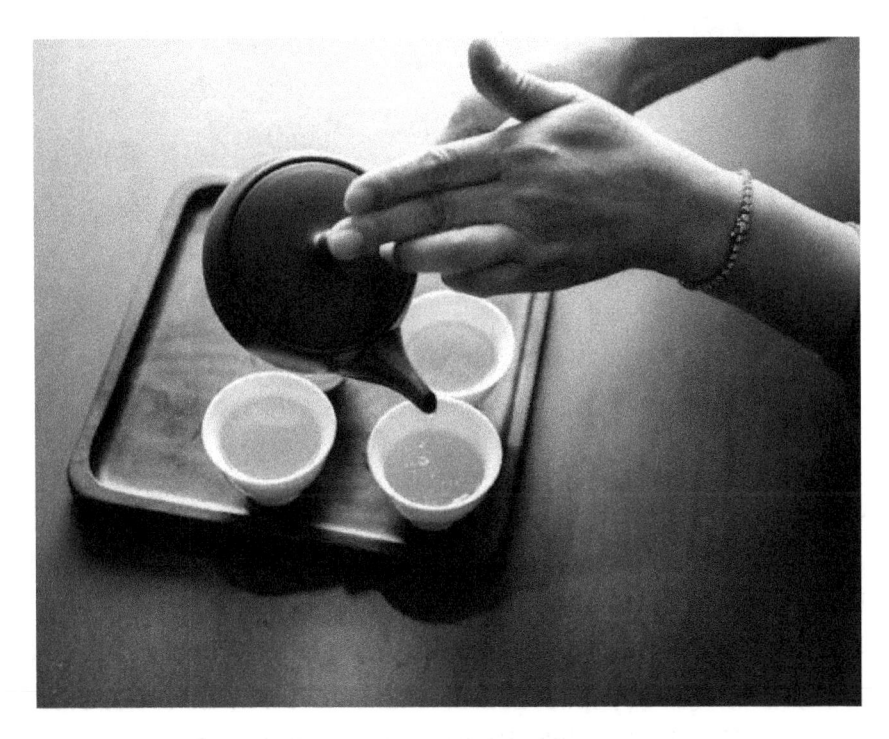

Green tea protects the skin from damage and aging. Green tea has potent compounds called catechins, a type of polyphenols having antioxidant and anti-inflammatory effects that improve your skin's health in several ways. Green tea helps lighten dark circles under your eyes as it is rich in vitamin K.

Drinking green tea every day could reduce redness from sun damage. Green tea is great for healing scars and blemishes and flushes out toxins. It also improves the moisture, roughness, thickness, and elasticity of the skin.

Avoid adding milk to your tea, milk could reduce the impact of green tea's antioxidants.

7. Oranges

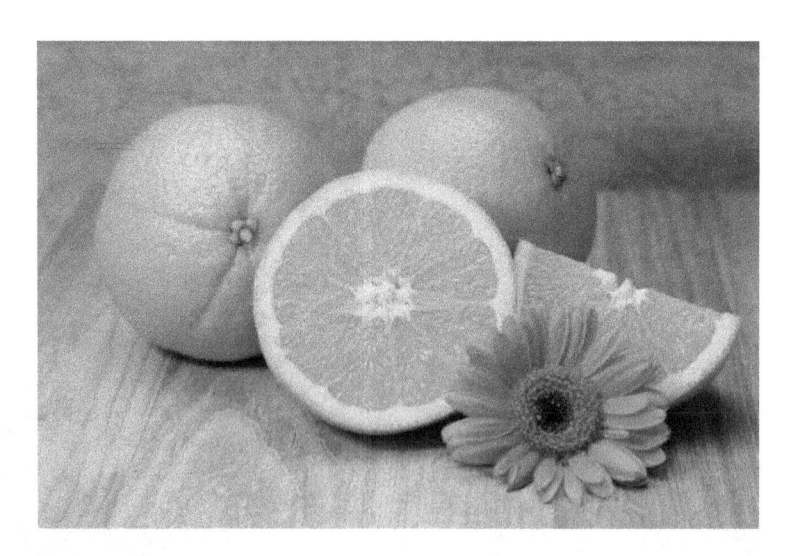

Oranges are citrus fruits packed with vitamin C, minerals, dietary fiber, which reduces wrinkles and age-related dry skin. Body needs vitamin C to produce collagen, a protein that keeps skin firm and fights the appearance of aging. Vitamin C boosts immunity, thereby protecting the skin from infections and diseases. Due to the high citric acid content, oranges help to dry out acne and aids in skin exfoliation, improving your skin's overall look.

Drinking orange juice regularly increases skin carotenoids, an antioxidant that can help protect the skin from harmful radiation, pigmentation and prevent inflammation. A single medium orange has more than enough of the daily recommended intake of vitamin C.

8. Papayas

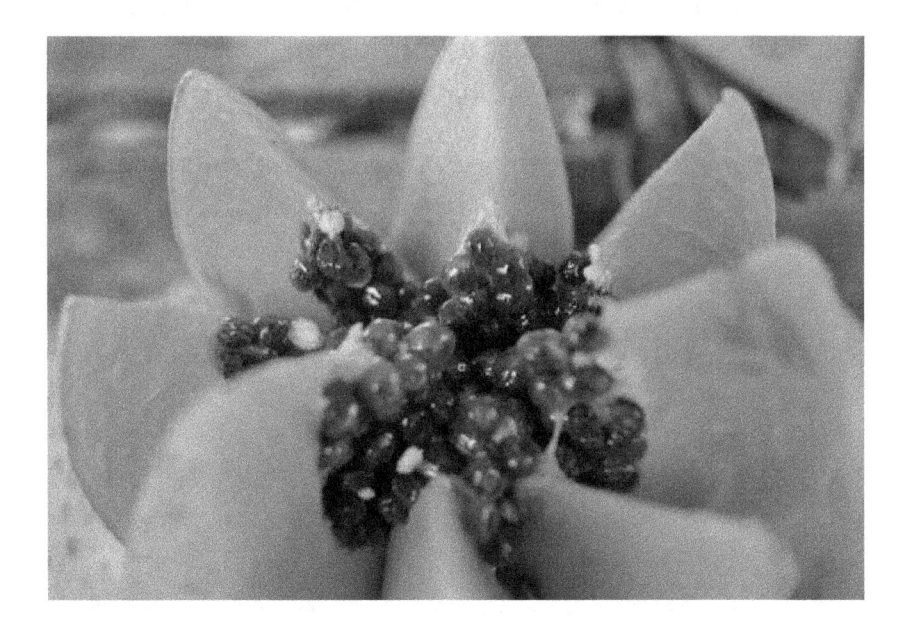

Papaya has skin-lightening properties that help clear blemishes and pigmentation. The delicious papayas contain enzymes papain and chymopapain, vitamins A, C, and B, and dietary fiber. Papaya improves bowel movement and digestion. This means you will be flushing out toxins that can prevent acne and pigmentation and help you get fresh and infection-free skin.

9. Avocados

Avocados help prevent sun damage while also strengthening and rejuvenating the skin. Avocados are high in monounsaturated fats and polyunsaturated fats, which are healthy fats. It is necessary to obtain a sufficient amount of these fats to keep your skin flexible and moisturized. These unsaturated fats benefit many functions in your body, including your skin's health. Avocados protect skin from oxidative damage caused by the sun, which can lead to signs of aging.

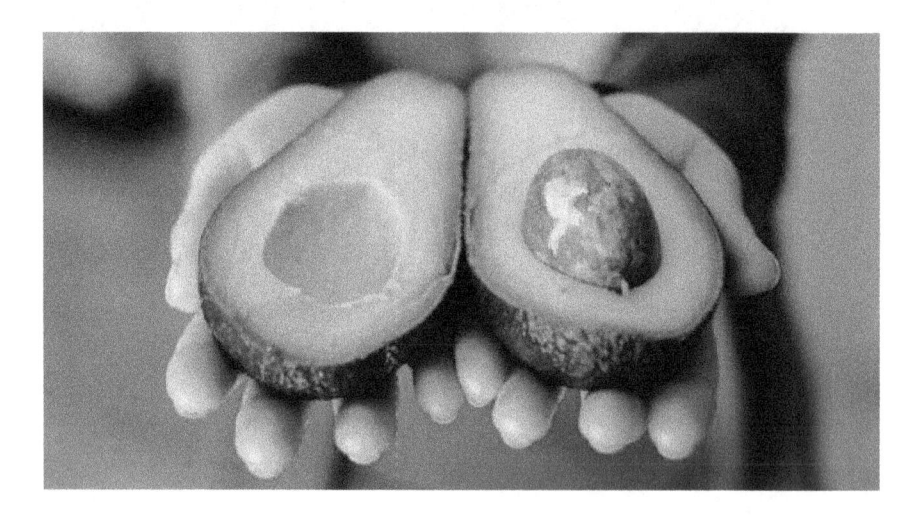

Avocados are high in vitamins A, C, E, K, B6, folate, niacin, pantothenic acid, riboflavin, choline, lutein, potassium, and magnesium. Getting enough healthy fats is important because they help maintain cell integrity and aid in healthy aging.

The antioxidants vitamins A and E guard against UV rays and keep skin moisturized. Avocados are also a good vitamin E source, an important antioxidant that protects your skin from oxidative damage. Skin needs Vitamin C to create collagen, which is the main structural protein that keeps your skin healthy.

10. *Olive Oil*

Olive oil consists mainly of oleic acid (approx 83%) monounsaturated fatty acids, which may play a role in the youth boost. The antioxidant polyphenols in olive oil help flush out the toxins and could also quench damaging free radicals.

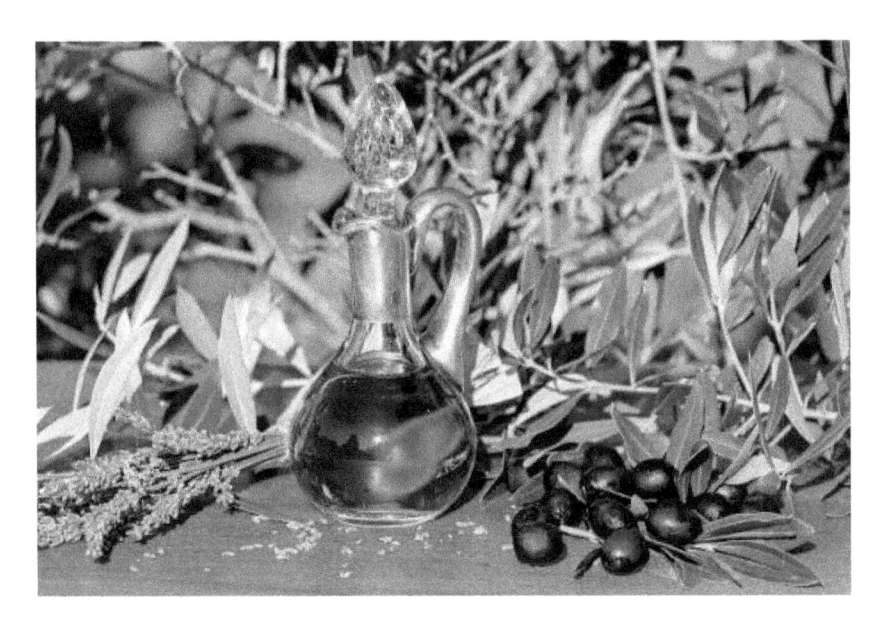

Olive oil is rich in vitamin E, which acts as an antioxidant that preserves your skin healthy and young. Topically applying olive oil can protect the skin from UV radiation and reduce the risk of skin cancer.

Conclusion

Who doesn't want clean, clear, and supple skin? Foods, as mentioned above, are readily available in the market. It would be a wiser decision to eat these foods instead of spending on cosmetics for better skin. Why go for a temporary solution for your skin when you can have permanent healthy, better-looking skin without any fuss. Think again!

CHAPTER 4

10 REASONS WHY FAT IS NOT THE ENEMY. THE TRUTH ABOUT FATS!

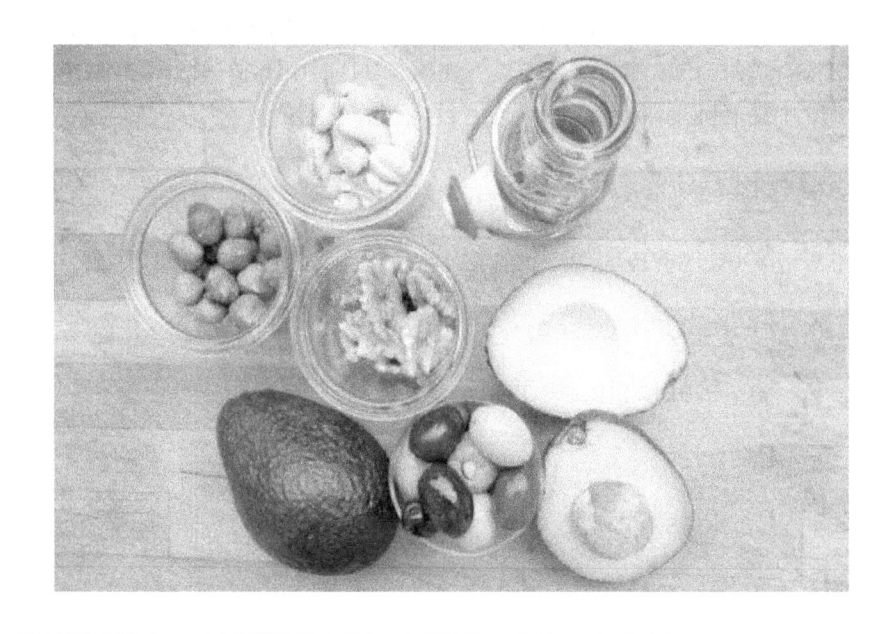

Did you know that the human brain is made up of nearly 60% fat? Fats are not something we should run from; our body needs a certain amount of fat to function at its best. Not all fats are bad; not all fats are good. Let's just quickly see which types of fat is our friend and which one is our enemy.

Types of Fat:

Trans Fats

Trans fats are the worst type of dietary fat. The hydrogenation process is used to turn healthy oils into solids to prevent them from becoming rancid, and a byproduct of this process is Trans fats. Trans fats do not have any health benefits, and there is no safe level of consumption. It is better to check the Nutritional Facts label on the packet of your packed food for any presence of trans fat. For every 2% of calories from trans-fat consumed daily, the risk of heart disease rises by 23%.

Food containing Trans Fat:

- Solid margarine
- French fries
- Vegetable shortening
- Pastries
- Cookies

Saturated Fats

They are solid at room temperature. A diet rich in saturated fats can increase total cholesterol, particularly harmful LDL cholesterol, that may cause blockages in arteries in the heart or elsewhere in the body. Saturated fat should be consumed in moderation, and it is recommended to limit the consumption of saturated fat to less than 10% calories a day.

Common sources of saturated fat:

- Whole milk
- Cheese
- Red meat
- Coconut oil
- Many commercially prepared baked goods

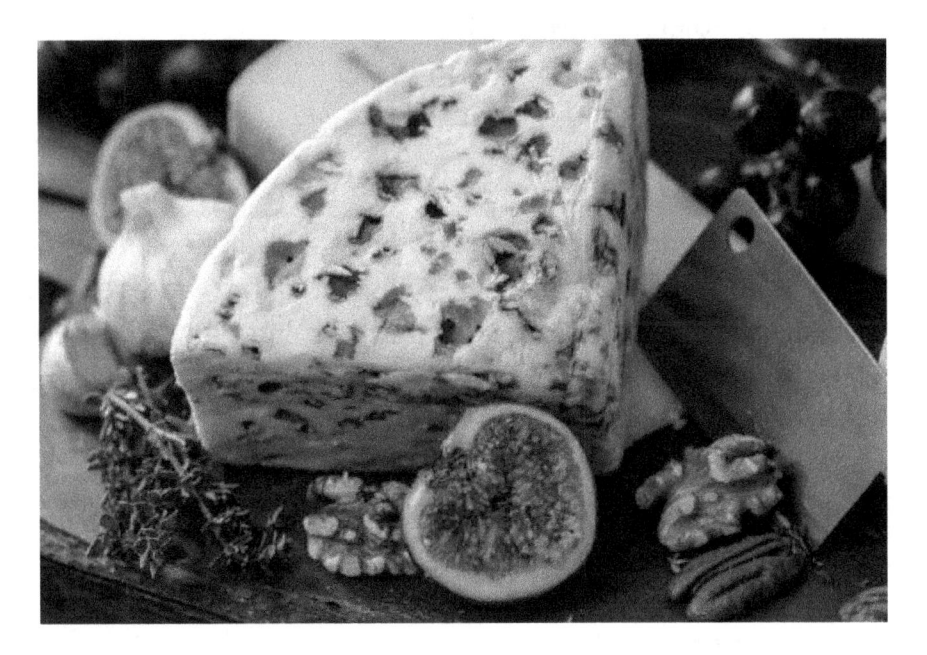

Unsaturated Fats

Monounsaturated and Polyunsaturated Fats

Monounsaturated and Polyunsaturated fats are healthy fats. They are liquid at room temperature and found in vegetables, nuts, and seeds. Polyunsaturated fats build cell membranes and the covering of nerves. They play an important role in blood clotting, muscle movement, and inflammation.

Good sources of monounsaturated fats are

- Extra virgin olive oil
- Sunflower oil
- Peanut oil
- Canola oil
- High-oleic safflower oil
- Avocado
- Nuts

Omega-3 fatty acids and omega-6 fatty acids are examples of polyunsaturated fats. Replacing saturated fats and refined carbohydrates with polyunsaturated fats can reduce harmful LDL cholesterol and improves the cholesterol profile. It also lowers triglycerides.

Good sources of omega-3 fatty acids include

- Flax seeds
- Chia seeds

- kidney beans
- Soybeans
- Walnut

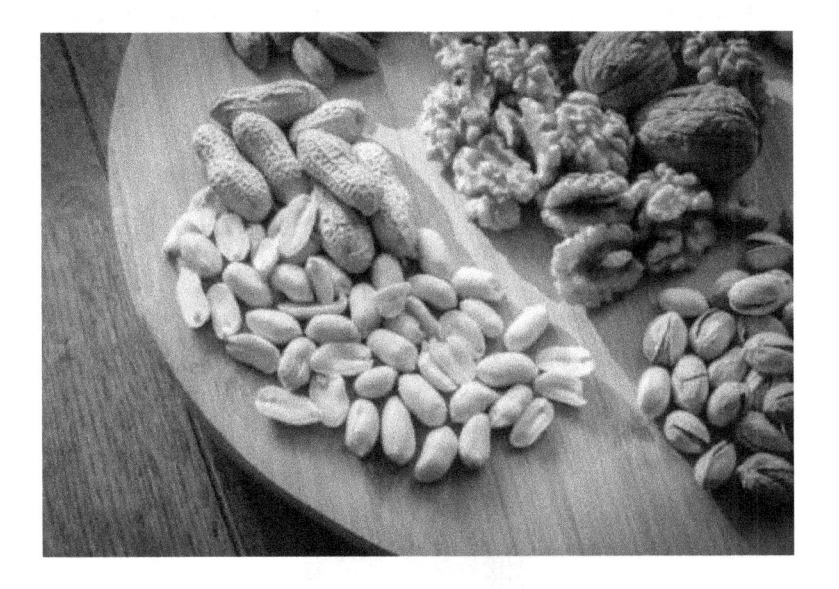

Omega-6 fatty acids have been linked to protection against heart disease.

Good sources of omega-6 fatty acids include

- Corn oil
- Sunflower oil
- Safflower oil
- Soybean oil
- Walnut

Below are the 10 reasons why fat is not the enemy:

1. Fat is Essential to Brain Health

Fat is essential to brain health. The brain is made of 60% fats, out of which a large chunk is docosahexaenoic acid (DHA) or Omega 3 fat.

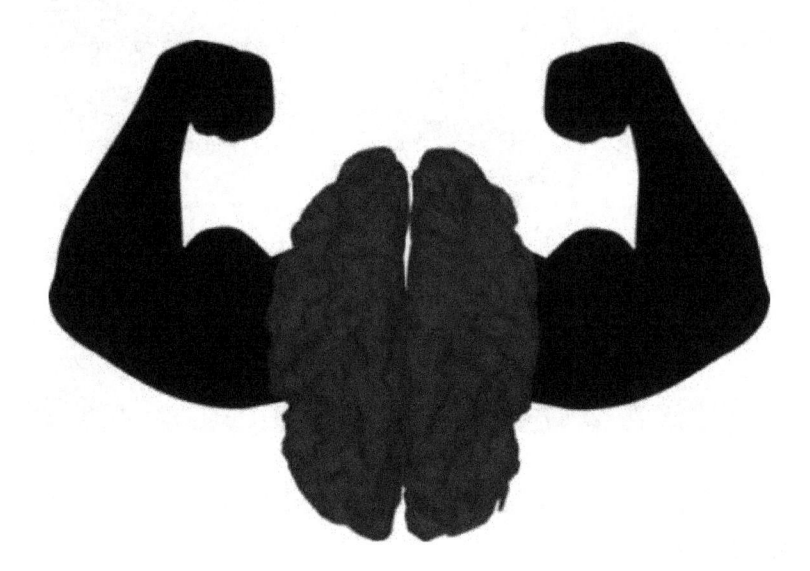

Essential fat-soluble vitamins such as A, D, E, and K are not water-soluble and require fat to get transported and absorbed in the body. These fat-soluble vitamins are crucial for brain health and many of your vital organs.

Vitamin D decreases susceptibility to Alzheimer's, Parkinson's, depression, and other brain disorders, and omega-3 is said to sharpen cognitive function and improve mood.

2. Fat for Better Skin

Fat forms cellular membranes and our skin is made up of a large number of cells. Without proper intake of fats, the skin can become dry and cracked, opening up ways for infections to enter your body.

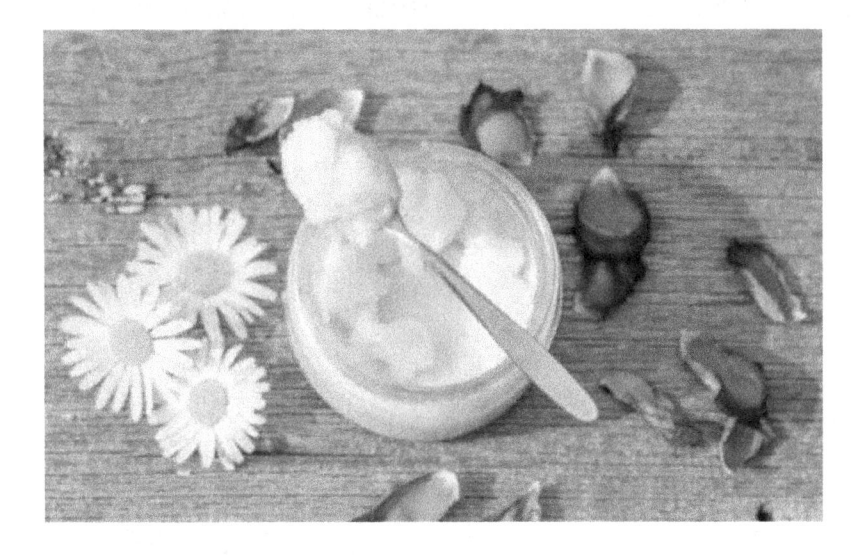

3. Fat Boosts Immune System

Fats are required for a healthy immune system. Saturated fats play an important role here, as adequate amounts will help the immune system recognize and then destroy foreign invaders.

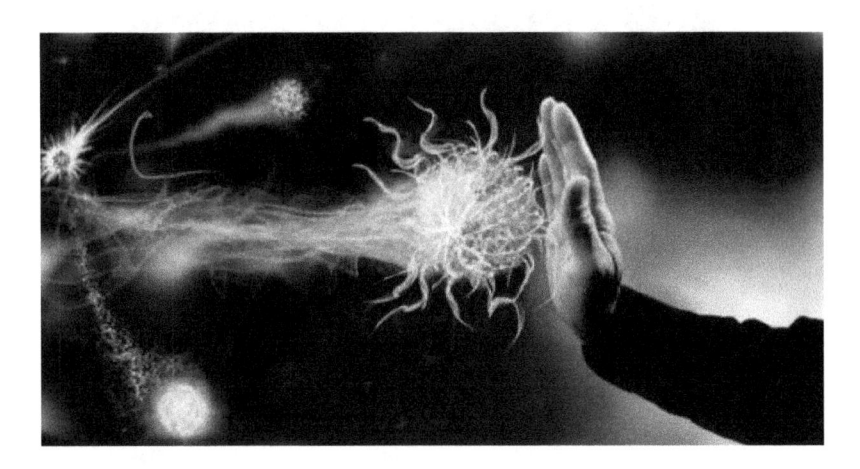

Read 10 Superfoods that Boost Immunity in the book Eat to Prevent and Controls Disease.

4. Fat Keeps Our Lungs Working Properly

Lungs are coated with a thin layer that is made up of 100% saturated fat. Fats are needed to protect this protective layer; Otherwise, it may result in breathing problems.

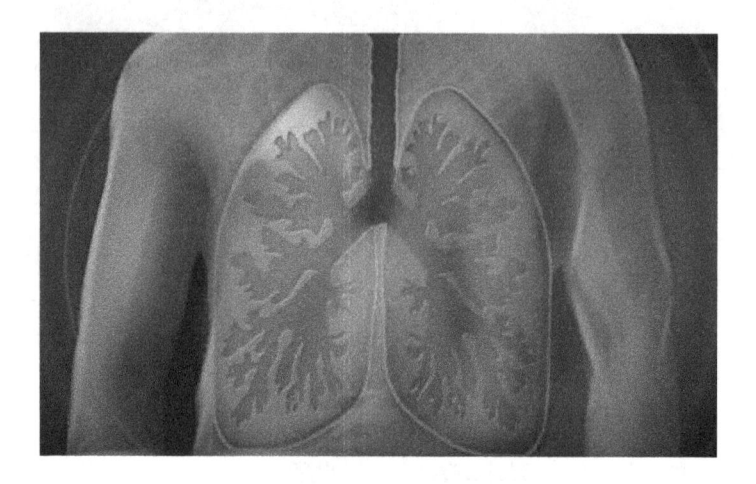

5. Fat is Good for Heart

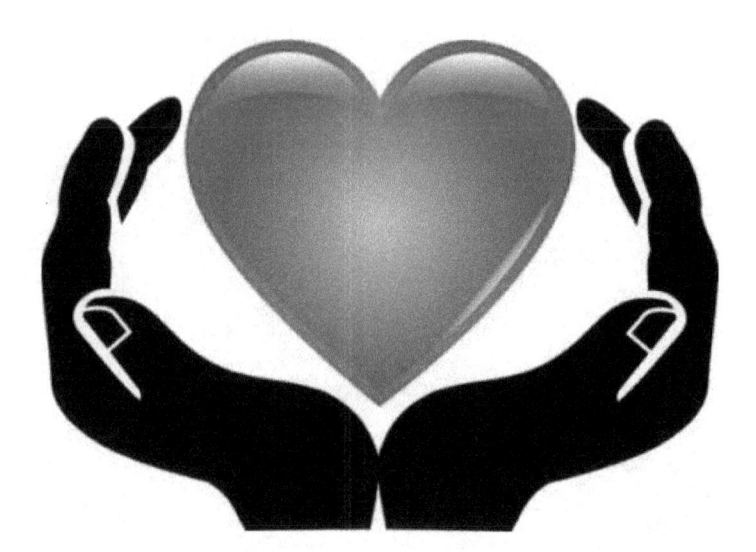

Unsaturated fats are healthy for the heart because they help lower blood pressure and slows the build-up of plaque in arteries by reducing triglycerides, a type of fat in your blood. Switching from saturated fats to polyunsaturated or monounsaturated fats can lower heart disease risk by up to 25%.

6. Fat Can Help You Lose Weight (Yes, you read it right)

Hungry cells cause weight gain. When you limit your calorie intake, your body goes into starvation mode, holding onto calories and storing fat.

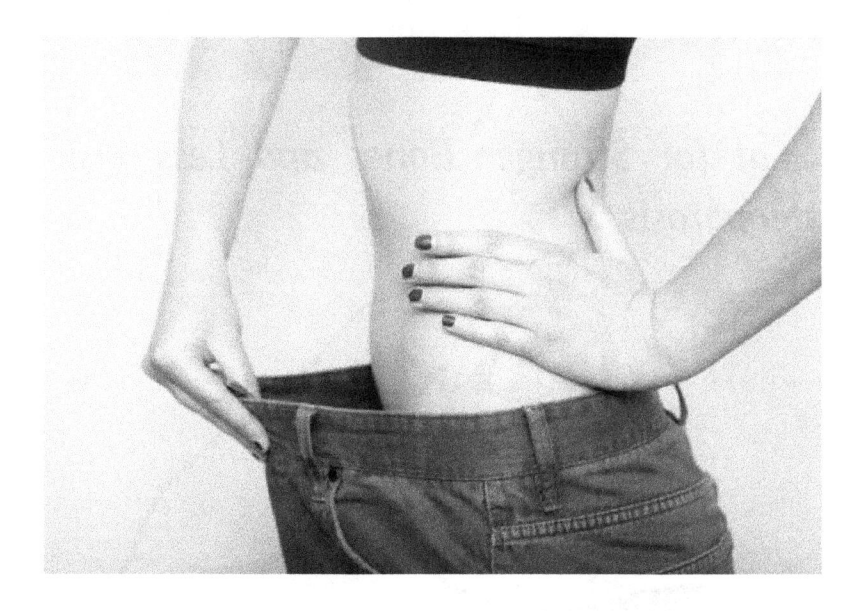

When you fuel your body with the right foods and enough healthy fats, your metabolism keeps running, and you are better at losing weight.

7. Fat for Proper Insulin Release

Saturated fats found in coconut oil help support proper nerve signaling by acting on signaling messengers. These messengers affect metabolism, as well as control the proper release of insulin.

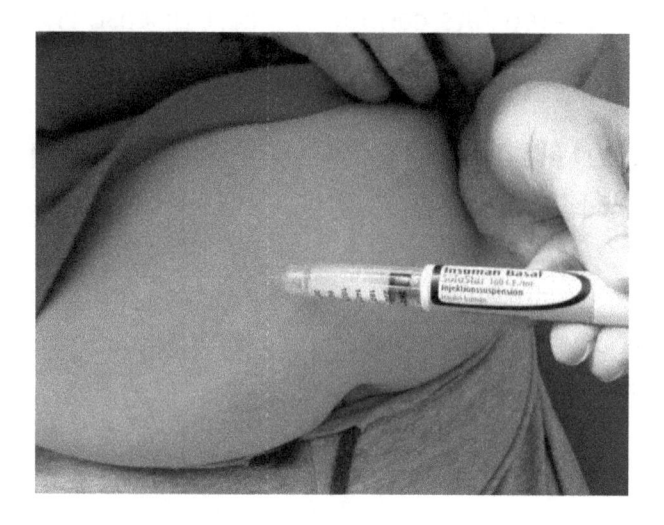

8. Fat for Stronger Bones and Less Risk of Osteoporosis

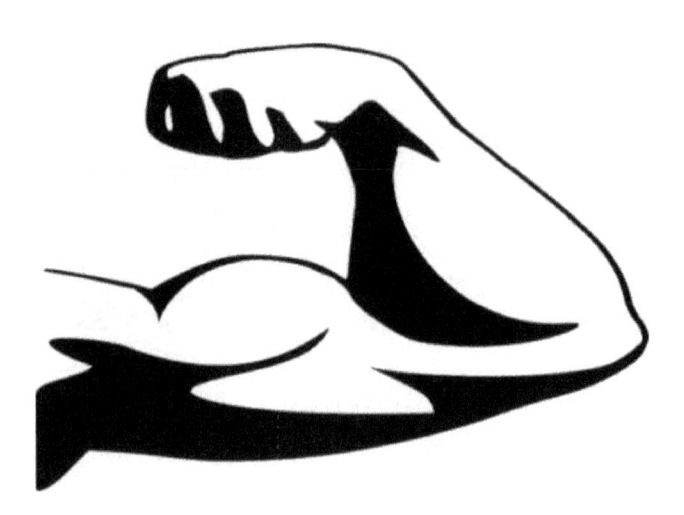

The important bone-building vitamins – Vitamin A, D, E, and K, are only fat-soluble, which means they are transported and absorbed using dietary fats. Fat is required for the metabolism of calcium.

9. Fat for Better Reproductive Health

Fats are the building blocks for healthy cell membranes and are important for hormonal health. Sex hormones – testosterone, estrogen, progesterone – are all made of cholesterol. Cutting way back on dietary fats can increase your risk of hormonal problems like hypothyroidism, menstrual irregularities, and low testosterone levels for men.

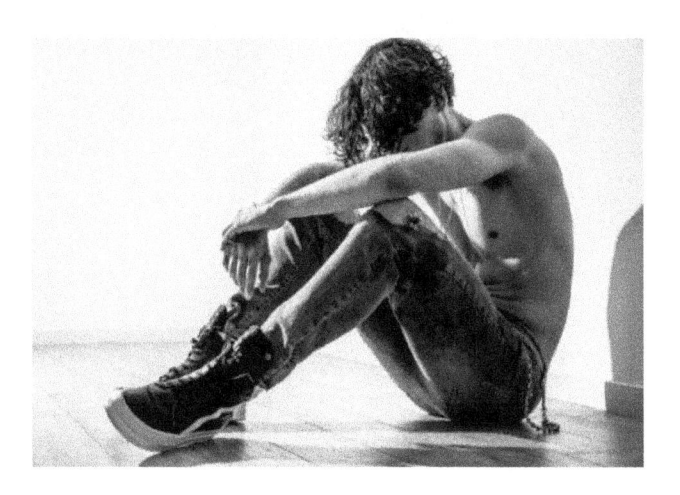

10. Fat for Better Eye Health

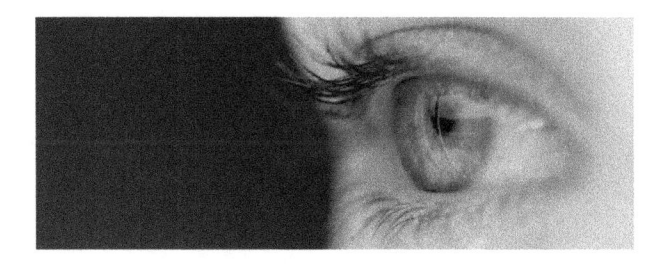

In dry eye disease, lack of tears leads to dryness, discomfort, and occasional blurry vision. Omega-3 fats help produce more tears and may benefit people with this condition. In addition, omega-3 fats help prevent diabetic retinopathy due to their anti-inflammatory properties.

Conclusion

No doubt not all fats are good for health, but at the same time, certain types of fats are essential for our health. Try to eat monounsaturated and polyunsaturated fats as much as you can (not beyond the limit) and limit your saturated fat consumption to less than 10%. Try replacing butter with extra virgin olive oil and French fries with nuts. These small changes in diet will result in a healthier and longer life.

CHAPTER 5

10 SMART WAYS TO LOSE WEIGHT WITHOUT DIETING

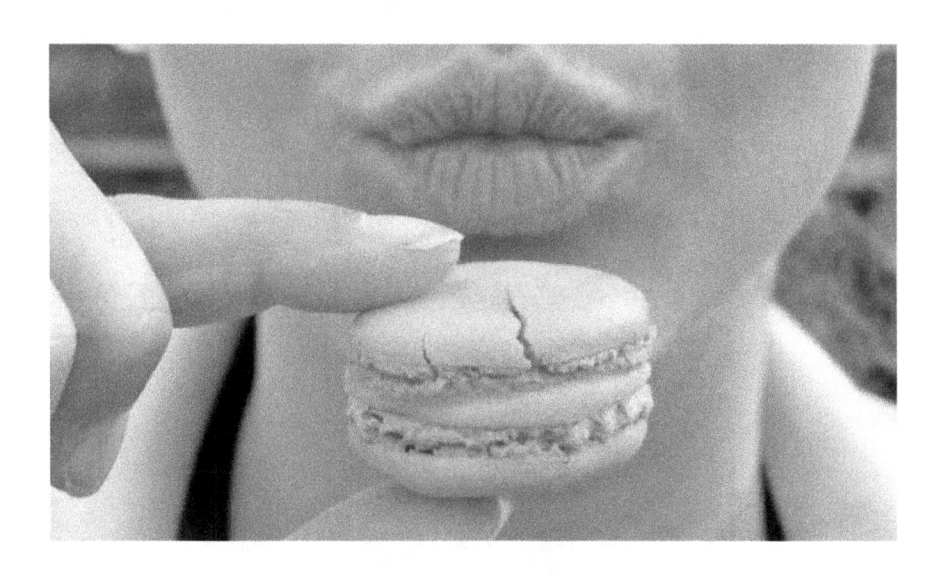

Diet plans can be challenging to stick to for prolonged periods. Imagine eating whatever you like, still not gaining an inch of extra fat. Yes, you read it right! There are other smart ways to lose weight without dieting. Implement the following tips in your life and maintain the desired weight you always dreamt of. These methods are the best-kept secrets for weight loss and work for everyone.

Read carefully the 10 smart ways to lose weight without dieting:

1. Hold Your Stomach In

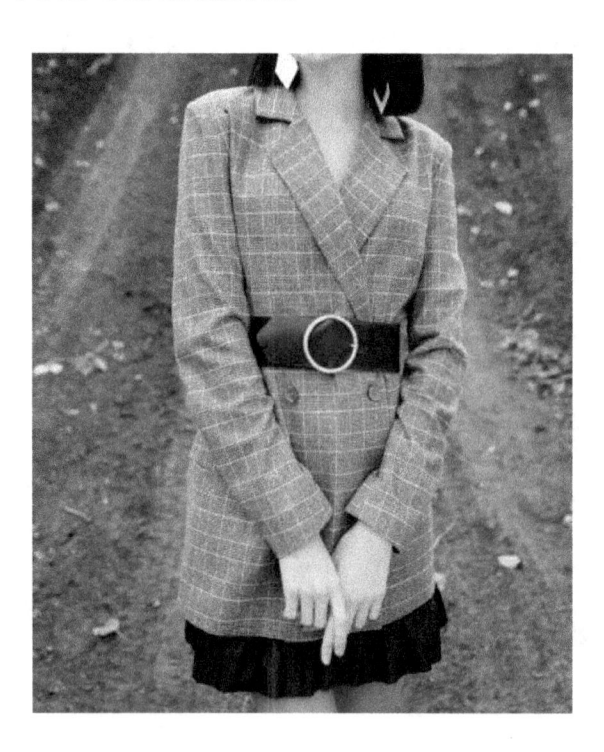

When you slightly tucked in your stomach while eating, you eat less. That doesn't mean you force yourself too much, but this trick always works. Wearing form-fitting clothes or wearing an outfit with a waistband serve as an alarm to prompt you to slow down. Not only while eating but in general hold your stomach in while sitting before the laptop or watching television, soon it will become a habit.

2. Laugh Out Loud

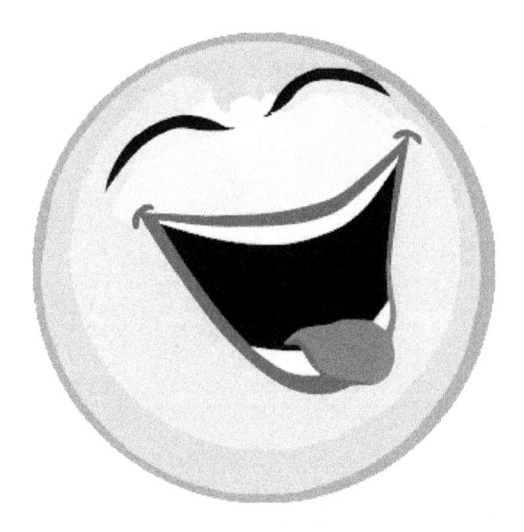

Laughter is a great antidote to stress. Laughing increases energy expenditure and increases heart rate by 10 to 20%. Laughter reduces cortisol levels, a stress hormone that lowers the metabolism and stores fat around the belly. This means laughter helps improve your metabolism naturally, which influences your body to burn more calories and lose weight.

3. Sleep Well

Sleep is like nutrition for the brain. Ideally, most people need 7 to 9 hours of sleep. Too little sleep triggers the stress hormone cortisol spike. Cortisol signals your body to conserve energy to fuel your waking hours. A lack of sleep may disrupt the appetite-regulating hormones leptin and ghrelin. Having these hormones fluctuate can increase your hunger and cravings for unhealthy food, leading to higher calorie intake. Lack of sleep and stress may increase the risk of several diseases, including obesity and type 2 diabetes.

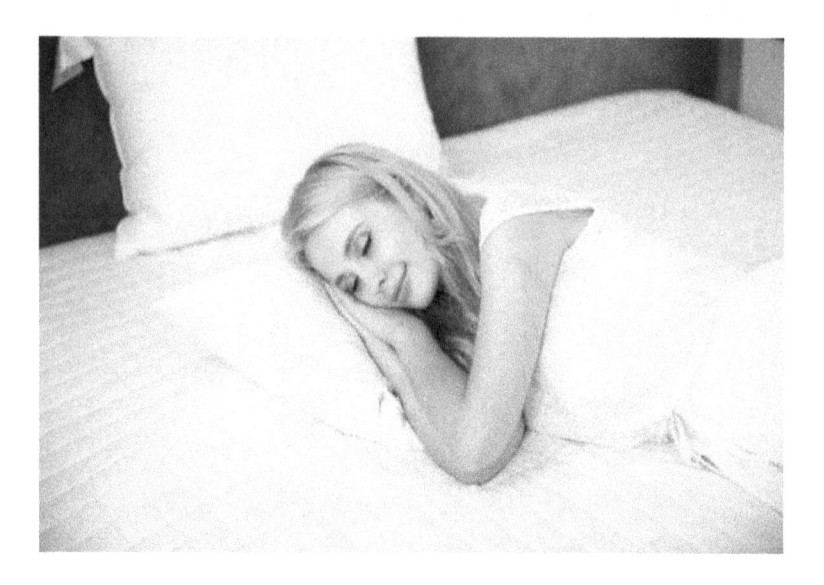

4. Eat Smaller Portions

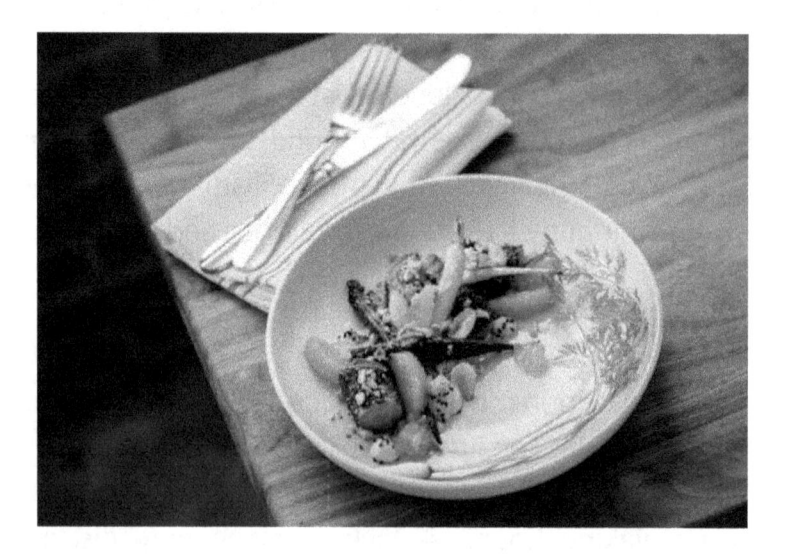

You can eat what you want, but the secret trick for losing weight is controlling the portion. Larger portions have been linked to weight gain and obesity because it encourages to eat more. To lose weight, you need to burn more calories than you consume, which inevitably means portion control. When you are eating out, sharing is caring. Try eating half or sharing the meal with a friend.

5. Eat Protein in Breakfast

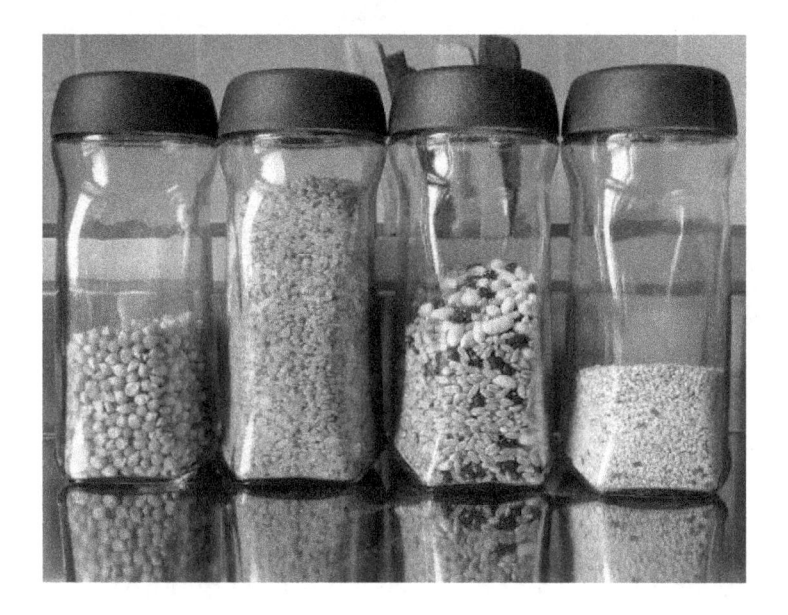

Eating protein in breakfast is important because it helps you feel fuller for longer. This is because protein affects several hormones, including ghrelin and GLP-1, that play a role in hunger and fullness.

Eating protein in breakfast slows down digestion, making you feel more satisfied by increasing feelings of fullness, reducing hunger, and eating fewer calories for the rest of the day. Some examples of protein-rich foods include lentils, quinoa, almonds, and Greek yogurt.

6. Take A Walk After Meal

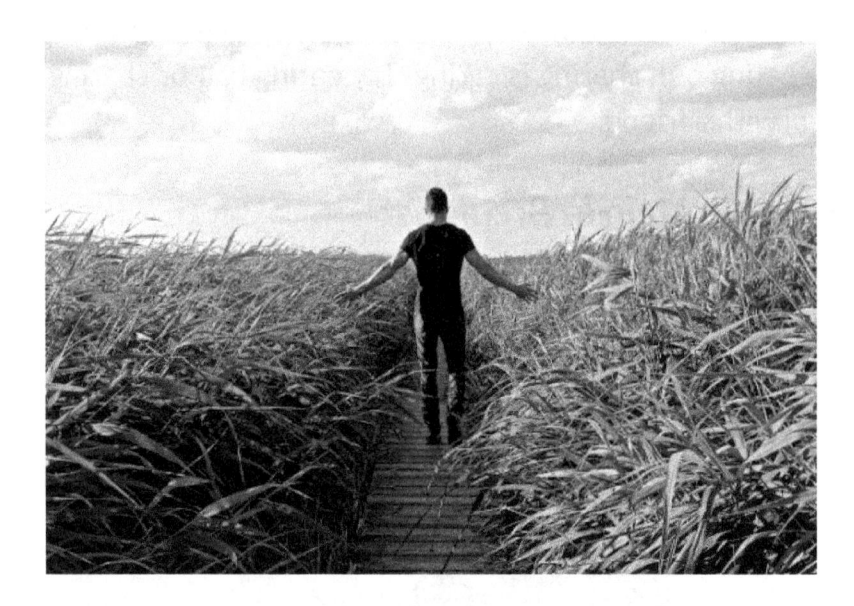

A brief walk shortly post-meal is a quick way to burn some calories and aid digestion. Your body digest food more quickly and efficiently when you take a walk after eating, as short as 15 min. In fact, it helps improve blood sugar levels, boost your energy, and burn calories. Walking for 30 minutes as soon as possible, just after lunch and dinner, leads to more weight loss than walking for 30 minutes, beginning one hour after a meal has been consumed.

7. Add Chili Peppers to Your Diet

Eating chili peppers can help you to lose weight by speeding up your metabolism and burning away fat. Capsaicin, a substance present in peppers, gives them their heat. The heat provided by capsaicin helps your body convert fat into heat and burn fat, resulting in weight loss.

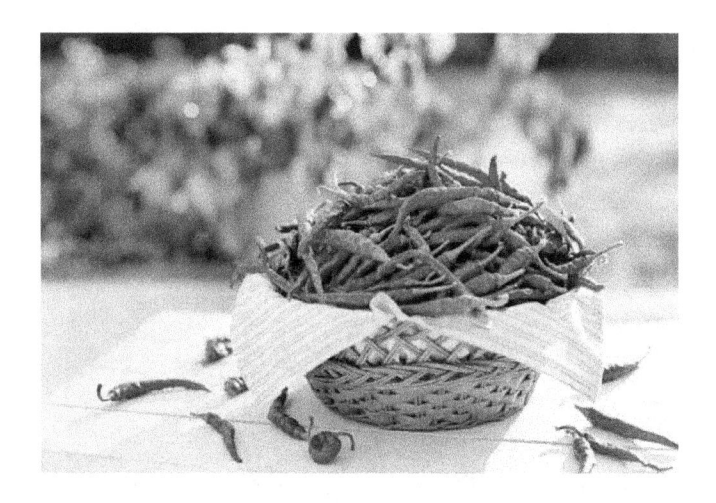

8. Eat Fiber-Rich Foods

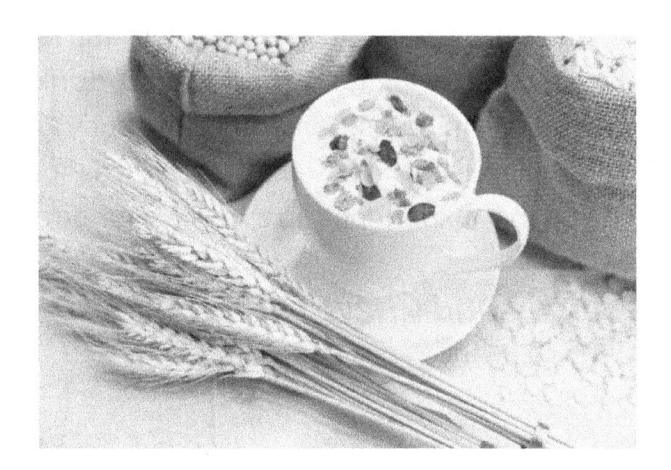

Eating fiber-rich foods helps you feel fuller for longer and increase satiety. Fiber has a Flush Effect, which means it helps reduce the absorption of calories from the food you eat. Fiber slows down the conversion of carbohydrates to sugar. This helps stabilize blood sugar levels and helps you lose weight. You can eat a lot of fiber-rich food without consuming a lot of calories. Some examples of fiber-rich foods include flax seeds, oats, beans, oranges, and Brussels sprouts.

9. Drink Water When You Crave for Snack

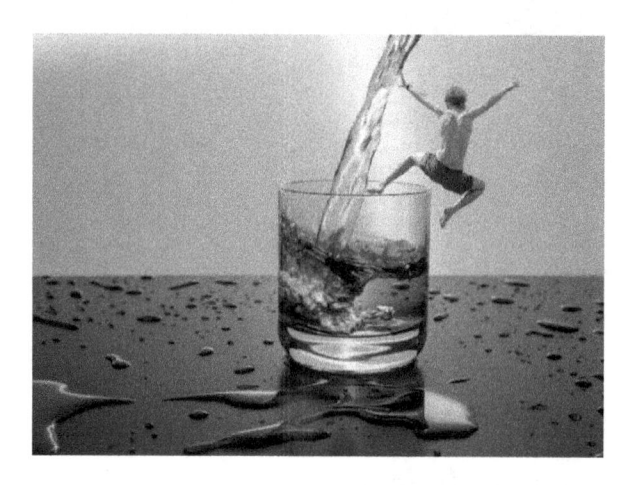

Water is an appetite suppressant. Drink at least 8 glasses (250 ml glass) of water in a day can help you eat less and lose weight. If you feel a sudden craving for a specific food, drink a glass of water and wait a few minutes. Sometimes our body gives a false alarm. If you replace sugar-loaded drinks such as soda or juice with water, you may experience an even greater effect.

10. Eat Slowly and Chew Thoroughly

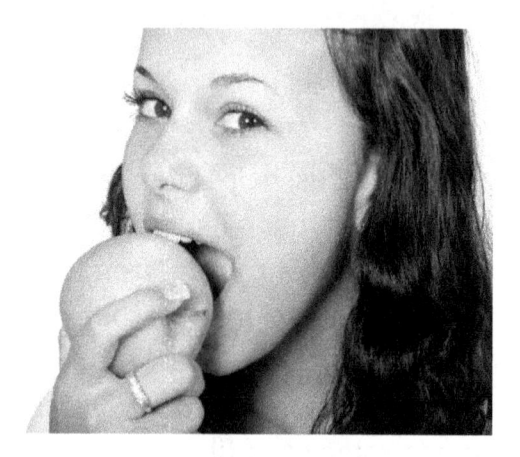

Your brain needs time to receive the fullness signals. It takes up to 20 minutes for your brain to get the signal that your stomach is full. Eating too quickly often leads to overeating. When you eat slowly, you consume less amount of food. Thoroughly chewing your food makes you eat more slowly. Chew your food at least 32 times. Chewing your food thoroughly also improves digestion and lets you lose weight faster.

Conclusion

A few simple lifestyle changes can have a massive impact on your weight over a long time. The best part of the above tips is that you don't need to give up completely your favorite food. However, adding exercise to these healthful habits can also improve a person's weight loss results. Don't take the burden on yourself by applying all the tips at once. Apply tips one by one, soon it will become your habit, and I bet you will never feel the need to go on a diet again in your life.

CHAPTER 6

10 REASONS WHY ALCOHOL IS A BIG NO NO!!!

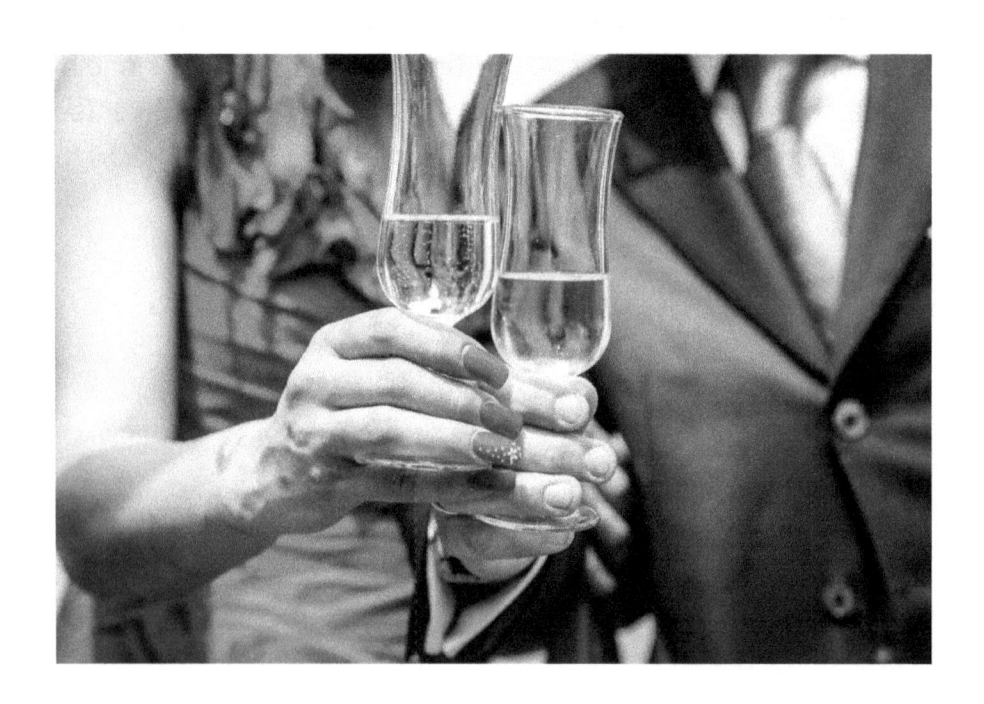

For many people, alcohol consumption has become a part of life. Alcohol is basically a chemical that can damage the body and may result in death. Still, drinking is considered socially acceptable in many parts because it is legal. Many people consider alcohol a stress reliever who wants to forget about the worries and tension of the day. However, as per a study, the fact is any amount of alcohol consumption is bad for health. If you are still not convinced, then read carefully below the most important reasons you should quit alcohol as early as you can.

Below are the Top 10 Reasons Why Alcohol is A Big No No:

1. Promotes Depression

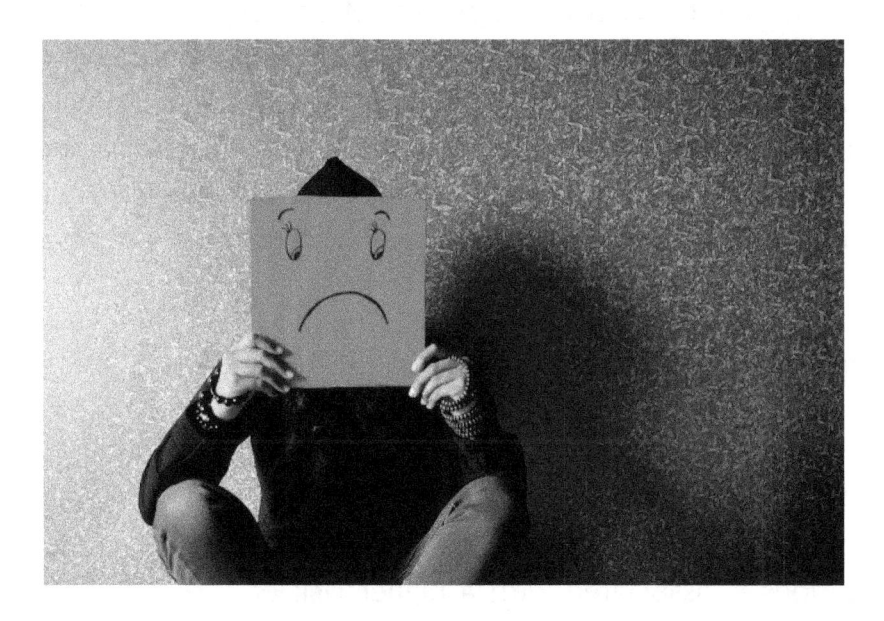

Are you worried about why you feel depressed all the time for every small issue? Alcohol is a direct central nervous system depressant that disrupts mood stability and promotes depression.

2. Brain Disorders

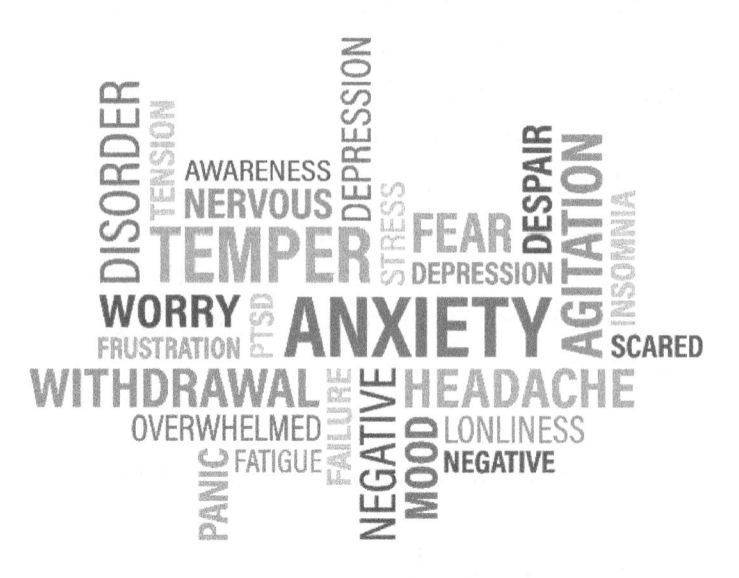

Alcohol interferes with the process of memory and affects the ability of new learning. Just one or two drinks are enough to cause slow reaction time, blurred vision, slow speech, impaired memory, and balance loss. These short-term effects disappear when you stop drinking alcohol, but prolonged alcohol consumption can cause neurological disorders that are severe and irreversible.

3. Cancer

International Agency for Research on Cancer (IARC) has classified alcoholic beverages as a Group 1 carcinogen (carcinogenic to humans). Drinking alcohol over extended periods is associated with a higher risk of certain types of cancer, including cancer of the mouth, throat, lung, esophagus, and breast. People who drink as well as smoke are at a higher risk of developing cancer. 3.6% of all cancer cases and 3.5% of cancer deaths worldwide are attributable to alcohol consumption (also known formally as ethanol).

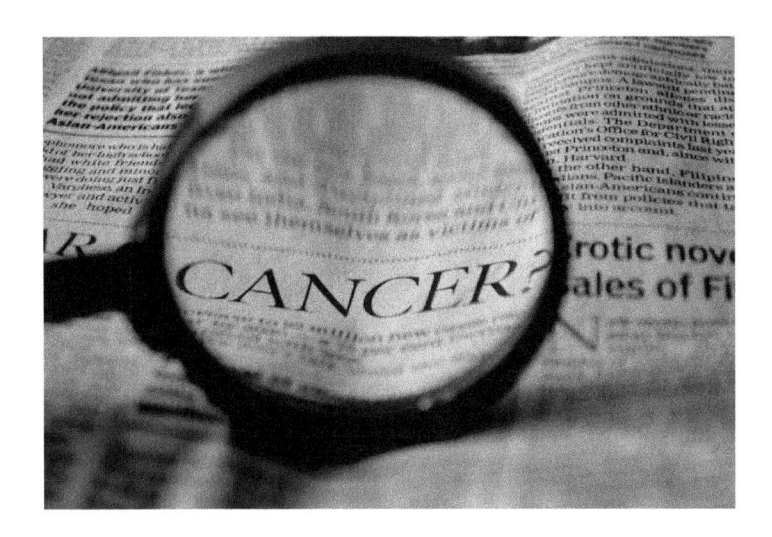

4. Weight Gain

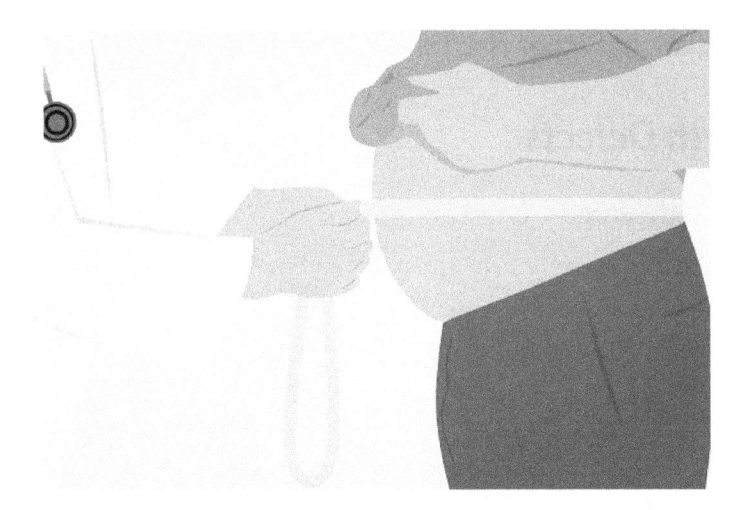

Alcohol can cause weight gain in many ways:

- It is high in calories.
- It stops your body from burning fat.
- It can make you feel hungry.
- It can lead to unhealthy food choices.

5. Risk of Injury

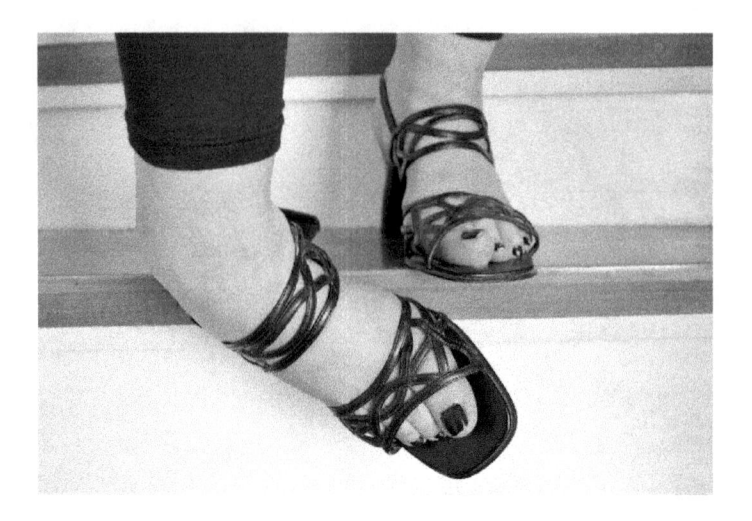

Alcoholic beverages slow the reaction time and impair judgment and coordination. People under the influence of alcohol are at higher risk for accidental injury.

6. Birth Defects

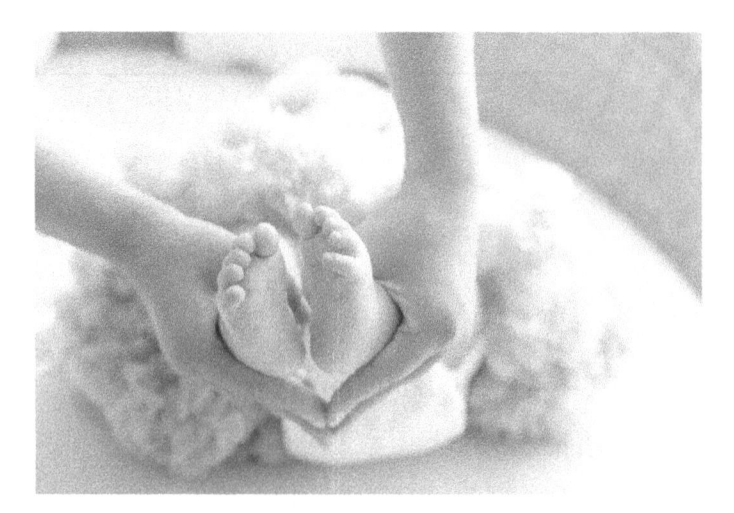

Pregnant women should not drink at all. Exposing the fetus to alcohol can cause defects of the brain, heart, and other organs in the baby. If a woman drinks alcohol while pregnant, the risk of giving birth to a child with fetal alcohol syndrome is very high. Fetal alcohol syndrome is a condition that affects the developing fetus. Children with fetal alcohol syndrome often have abnormal facial characteristics, stunted growth, organ defects, brain damage, and poor coordination. Fetal alcohol syndrome cannot be cured. Once the damage has been done to a child, he or she must suffer for life.

7. Cirrhosis of the Liver

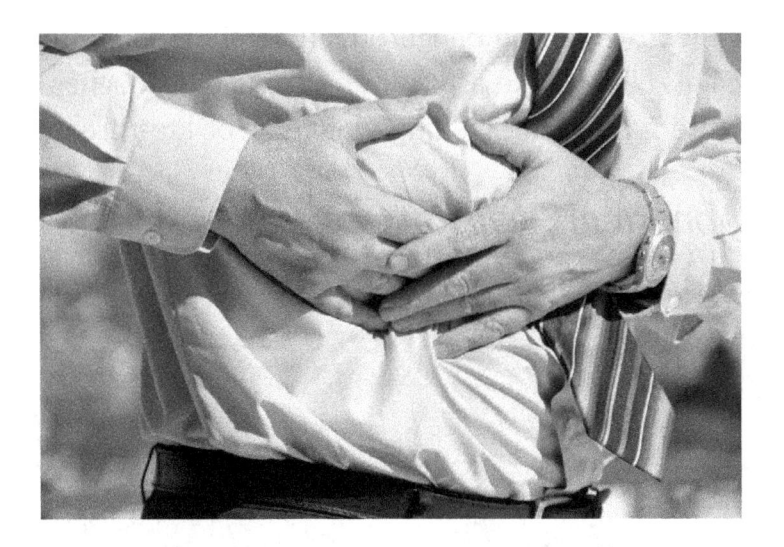

Alcohol can lead to permanent organ damage. Liver cirrhosis can be fatal because the damaged liver cannot perform the essential processes required to keep the body functioning optimally. Cirrhosis affects the liver's ability to convert food into energy and prevent the removal of toxins from the body. When you have cirrhosis, your liver contains scar tissue that reduces blood flow through the organ. As a result, the liver cannot work effectively.

8. Serious Chronic Diseases

Long-term alcohol consumption can raise blood pressure and increase heart attack risk. Drinking too much alcohol can cause liver cirrhosis (damage to liver cells) and pancreatitis (inflammation of the pancreas).

9. Drug Interaction

Alcohol interferes with the therapeutic effect of the prescribed medication, including anti-depressant and anti-anxiety medications. It can be dangerous in combination with other medicines. Never take aspirin for alcoholic headaches. It can cause internal gastric bleeding, which can be life-threatening.

10. Abnormal Sleep Pattern

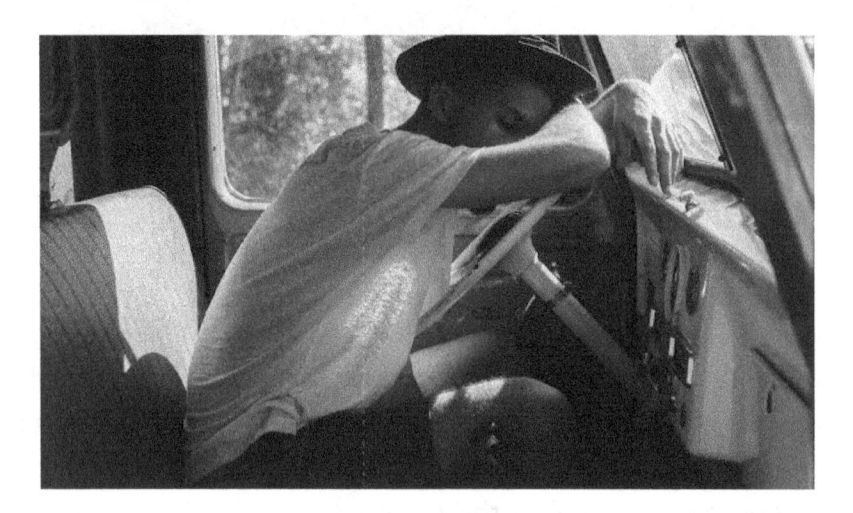

Alcohol interrupts the normal sleep pattern, which affects energy, mood, anxiety level. You feel tired all day.

My Thoughts

It is a misconception that you can enjoy your life only with a glass of alcoholic drink. It is a human tendency to follow what we see. It is not entirely our fault as we often see alcohol in movies and serials as a fun factor of life. They portray the most dangerous substance- alcohol as a cool thing or as a status symbol. But we should never forget that movies and serials are the pure art of fiction and have nothing to do with real life. Being a scientist, I have worked closely with alcohol. Alcohol is just another chemical substance that we use in minimal quantity to prepare tablets and capsules to treat a particular disease. We use it in lesser quantity because we know how dangerous alcohol is for the human body. You only live once; It is better to live your life disease-free, frustration-free, and depression-free. This is your fundamental right, do not let alcohol steal your basic living rights.

CHAPTER 7

10 REASONS YOU SHOULD START EATING ALMONDS EVERY DAY

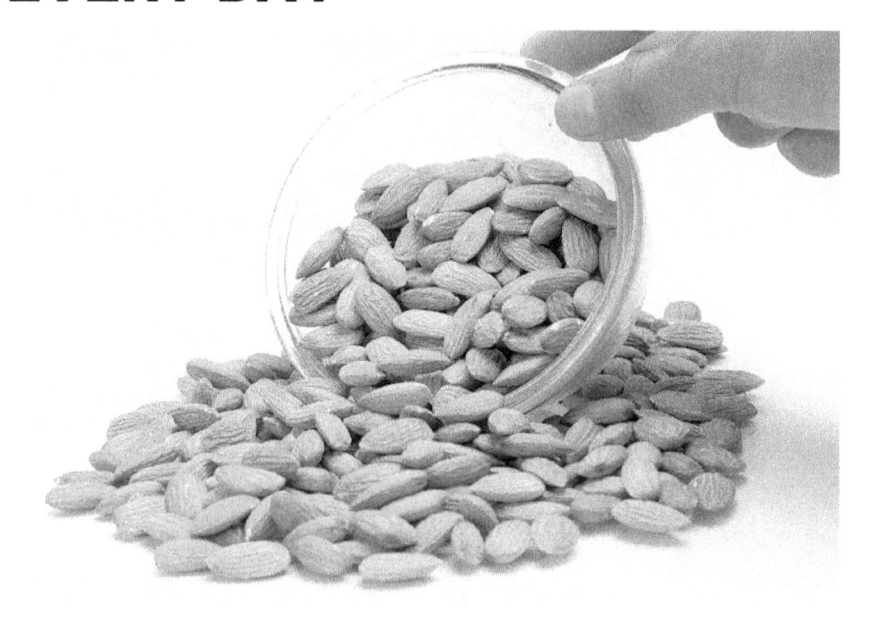

Almonds are among the healthiest of tree nuts. Natural, unsalted almonds are nutritious snacks loaded with minerals with plenty of health benefits. Just a handful of almonds (10-15 kernels) a day helps promote heart health, skin and hair health and prevent weight gain, and it may even help fight diseases like Alzheimer's and diabetes.

Types of almonds:

Bitter: These almonds are used for making (almond) oil, which has multiple benefits.

Sweet: Sweet almonds are edible.

Below are 10 Reasons You Should Start Eating Almonds Every Day:

1. Almonds Improve Skin Health

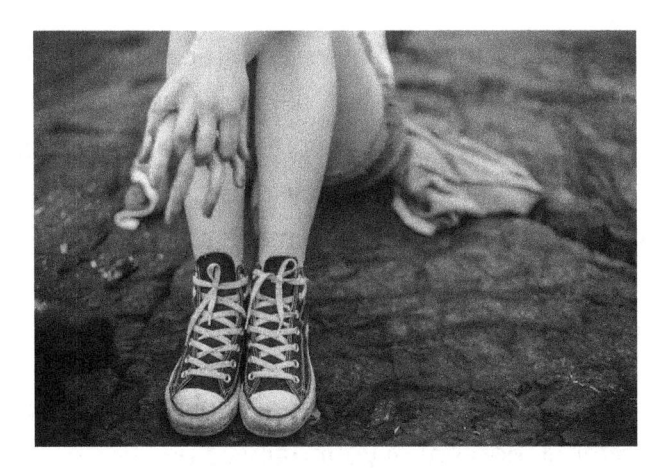

Want to have glowing, healthy skin? Eat almonds! Almonds are a great source of vitamin E and antioxidants, which fight free radicals and reduce inflammation, preserving your skin healthy and young. People with dermatitis should eat almonds daily. Antioxidants in almonds can fight the damage produced by UV rays, pollution, and a poor diet on the skin. Almonds fight against aging, malnourished skin and prevent skin cancer.

2. Almonds Maintain a Healthy Brain Function

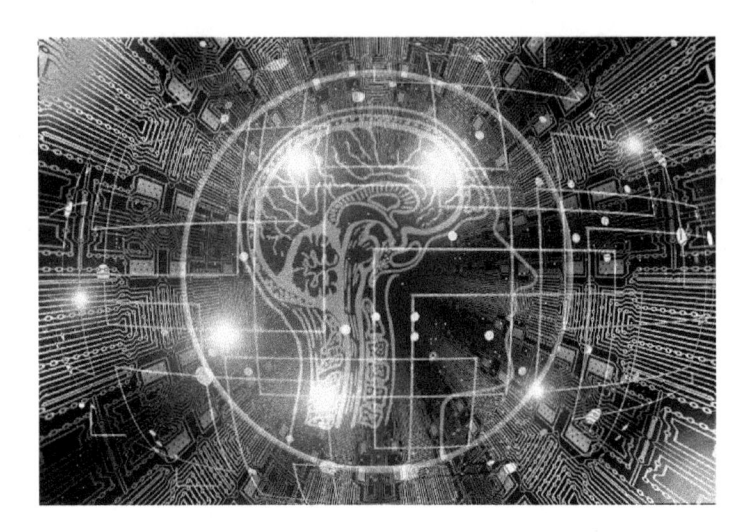

Almonds are rich in riboflavin and L-carnitine. These two substances prevent cognitive decline and support healthy neurological activity, reducing the brain's inflammatory processes. Eating almonds every day can prevent cognitive diseases like dementia and Alzheimer's disease.

3. Almonds Improve Hair Health

Almonds are absolutely bursting with biotin. A single serving contains over 50 percent of your daily value. Biotin (also known as vitamin H) helps many bodily processes, but perhaps its most prominent role is to aid in forming healthy hair. Biotin deficiency can lead to an unhealthy scalp and brittle, thinning hair. Since just a single serving of almonds contains over half your daily requirement, they're a fantastic food for keeping hair strong, healthy, and beautiful.

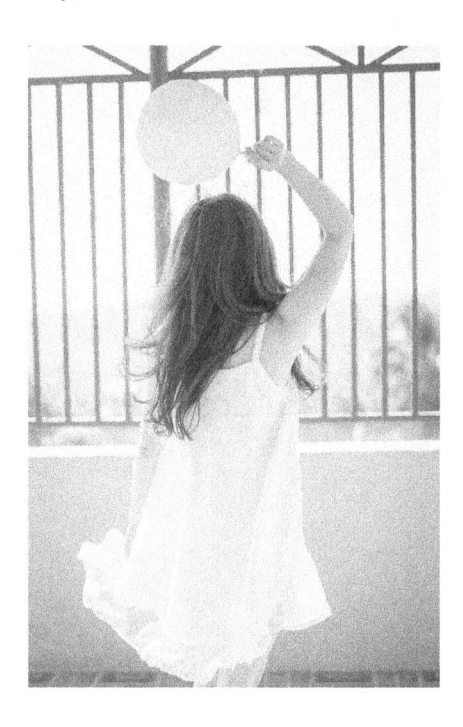

*Read 10 Most Important Nutrients for Hair Health in the book Secret of Healthy Hair.

4. Almonds Keep Heart Healthy and Prevent Heart Attacks

Almonds have high levels of monounsaturated and polyunsaturated fats. Also known as "good fats," they have been shown to have a significant positive impact on cholesterol. A better cholesterol profile greatly reduces the risk of blocked arteries, the biggest culprit behind heart attacks and strokes. Eating more almonds equals a healthier heart.

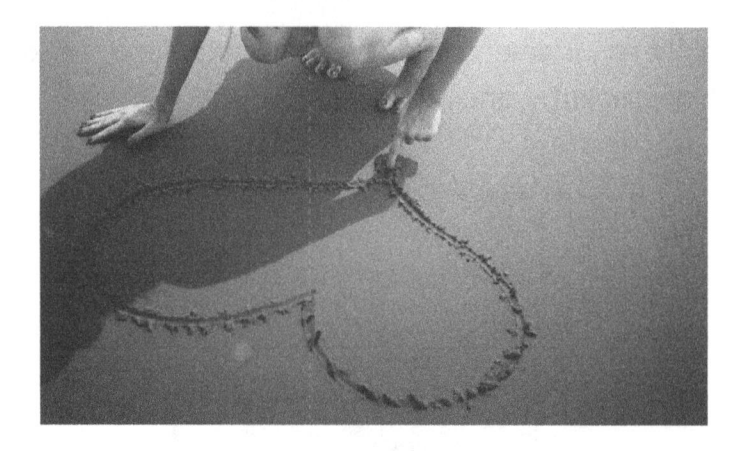

5. Almonds for Weight Loss

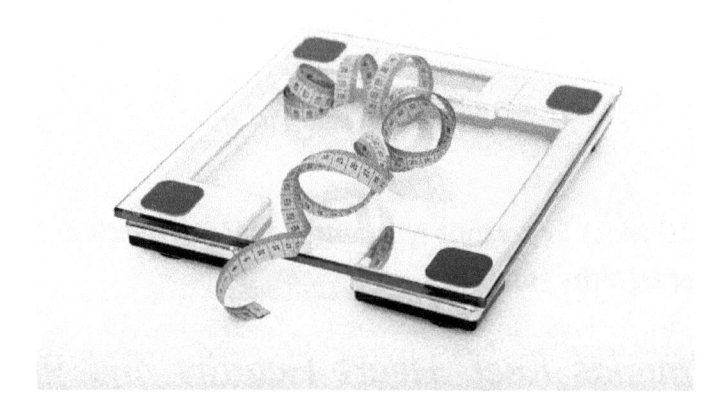

Almonds are packed with a lot of fiber and protein content which takes a longer time to digest, which results in a fuller stomach and lesser cravings. Plus, protein helps in the development of lean muscle mass. Almonds are a perfect low-carb snack and ideal for those who are on a low-carb diet.

6. Almond Benefits Blood Pressure Levels

Almonds fend off magnesium deficiency. Magnesium deficiency is strongly linked to high blood pressure. If you do not meet the dietary recommendations for magnesium, adding almonds to your diet could have a huge impact. The magnesium in almonds may help lower blood pressure levels. High blood pressure is one of the leading drivers of heart attacks, strokes, and kidney failure.

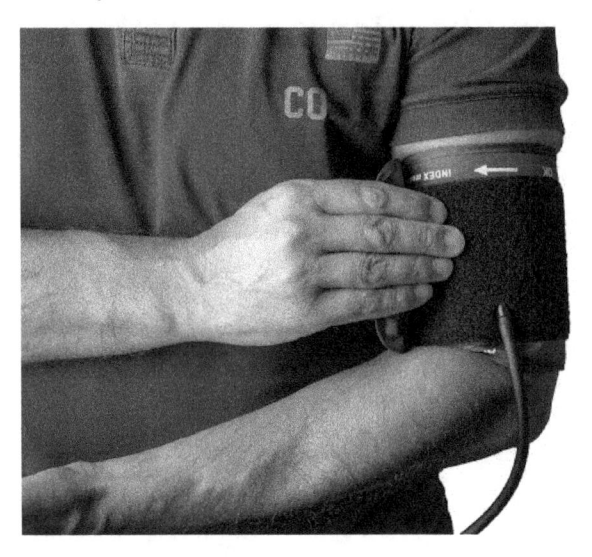

7. Almond Increase Digestion and Metabolism

Almonds are good for digestion. Along with being high in vitamin E and other minerals, almonds are now believed to increase good bacteria in the gut. Eating almonds can help improve digestive health. Almond milk has secret traces of digestive-enhancing fiber. Thus, almond milk reduces the problem of indigestion to a great extent. Increased digestion removes unwanted and unhealthy toxins from the human body system. It further increases the metabolic rate.

8. Almonds Prevent Cancer

Almonds are an excellent source of vitamin E, phytochemicals, and flavonoids, which control the progression of breast cancer cells. The fibers in almonds help detox the body. This enables food to move more efficiently through the digestive system. This process cleanses the digestive system, thus reducing the risk of colon cancer.

9. Almonds Strengthen Bones and Teeth

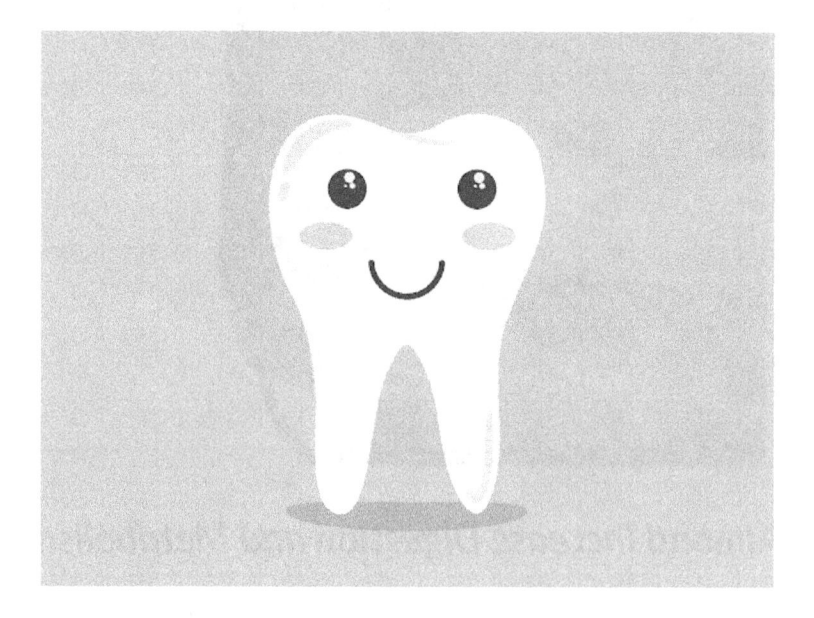

Almonds contain about 200 milligrams of the recommended daily dose of calcium. They also contain a whole host of nutrients — fiber, manganese, phosphorus, vitamin E — that reduce osteoporosis, strengthen teeth, improve mineral density of bones, and strengthen the skeletal system.

10. Almonds Prevent Birth Defects

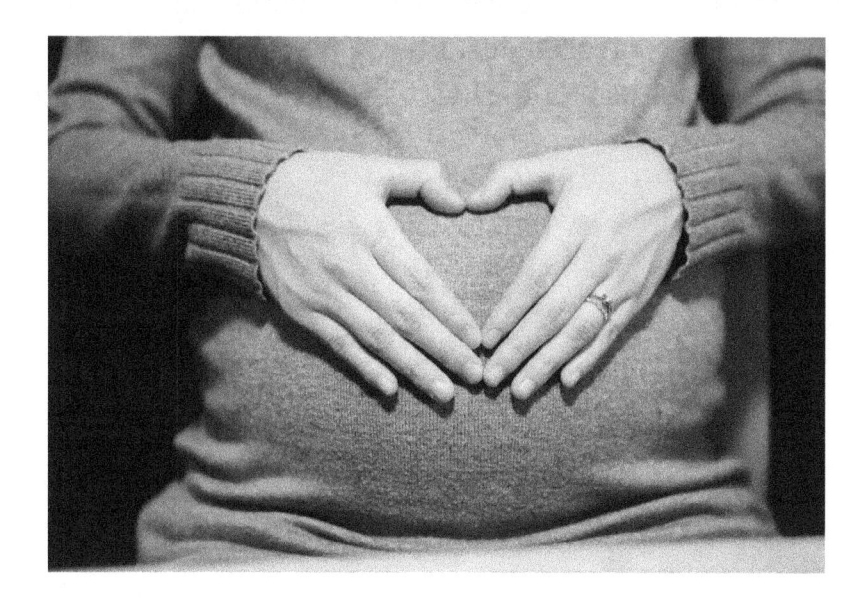

Folic acid in almonds protects the baby while still in the womb from neural tube defects. Folic acid has a significant function in healthy cell growth and tissue configuration and is, therefore, very important for the healthy development of the fetus. It also helps with the development of the nervous system and the bones.

Conclusion

One should eat soaked almonds as soaking almonds neutralize enzyme inhibitors, thus aiding digestion. Soaking almonds helps to reduce the phytic acid in the outer layer of almonds. The outer layer of almond bran can block calcium absorption and affect magnesium, iron, copper, and zinc absorption. Soaked almonds have higher B Vitamins. They help with the breakdown of gluten, which neutralizes toxins in colons and makes proteins more available for absorption. It should also be kept in mind that almonds contain calories and should be consumed in controlled quantities. Excessive consumption of almonds can be bad for the heart as well as your body weight.

CHAPTER 8

10 SMART WAYS TO INCORPORATE PUMPKIN INTO YOUR DIET

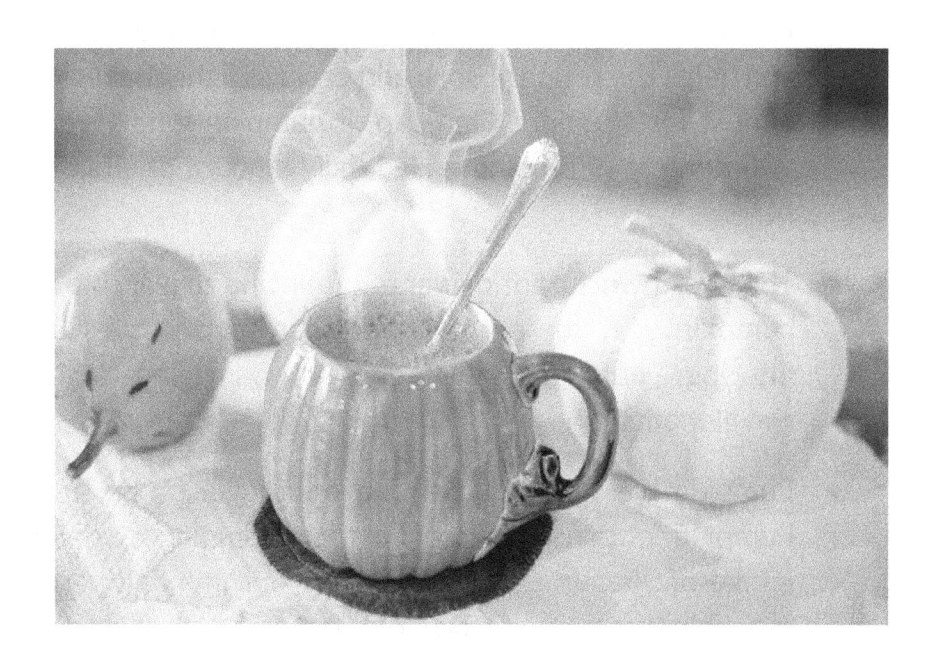

When I was a kid, my Mom used to chase me to make me eat pumpkin subji (curry) along with a long lecture on the benefits of the pumpkin, but as a kid, I was not a fan of pumpkin. Yes, we all have been gone through this. I wish someone had told my Mom the smart ways to incorporate pumpkin into the diet like I am telling you today.

Before going into more detail, let's first see why pumpkin is so important to eat, especially if you are a student.

Benefits of Pumpkin:

- Pumpkin is high in vitamins and minerals and low in calories as it's 94% water which makes it a weight-loss-friendly food.

- Pumpkin is rich in beta-carotene that converts into vitamin A in the body. Vitamin A is essential for eyesight and helps the retina absorb and process light, making it a must for students. One cup of pumpkin fulfills over 200 percent of recommended daily amount of vitamin A.

- The two powerful antioxidants, lutein and zeaxanthin in pumpkin, play the part of sunscreen for the eyes by filtering out the high-energy damaging light wavelengths.

- Pumpkin has antibacterial and antifungal properties. Pumpkin contains 20 percent of the recommended daily intake of vitamin C, which boosts your immunity and may help you recover from colds faster.

- Research suggests that a diet rich in beta-carotene can reduce the risk of prostate cancer.

Now we know how much pumpkin is important to our health. Below are 10 smart ways to incorporate pumpkin into your diet:

10 Smart Ways to Incorporate Pumpkin into Your Diet:

1. Pumpkin Oats Cake

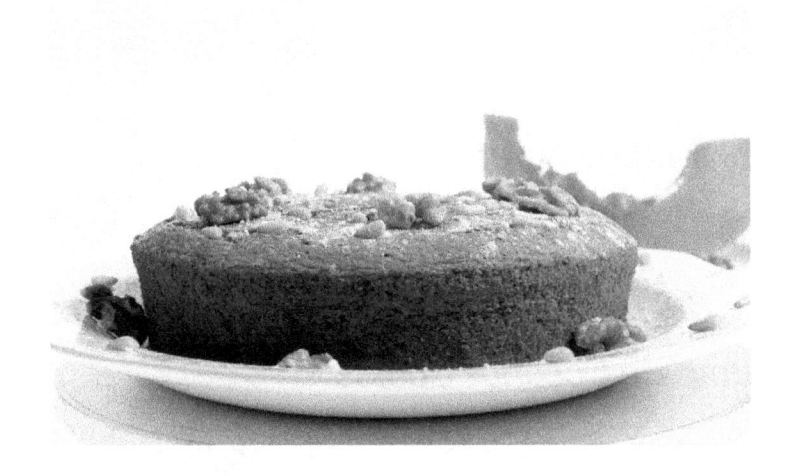

When you can't get your mind off sweet, try this healthier option. Instead of your regular cake, enjoy pumpkin and oats cake. Spiced with nutmeg and honey, 2-3 slices of this cake are enough to provide the required vitamin A for the entire day.

2. Pumpkin Halwa

Give *gajar ka halwa* a rest for some time, and try this exotic pumpkin halwa this time. Top it off with some roasted desiccated coconut, almonds, and enjoy this dessert.

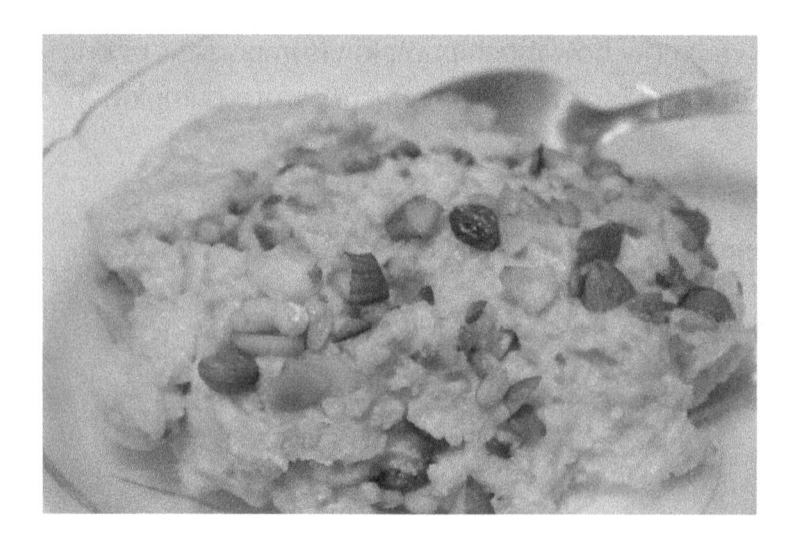

3. Roasted Pumpkin

Replace your regular French fries with roasted pumpkin. Bake pumpkin pieces and spice them up with peri-peri masala.

4. Pumpkin Coconut Cookie

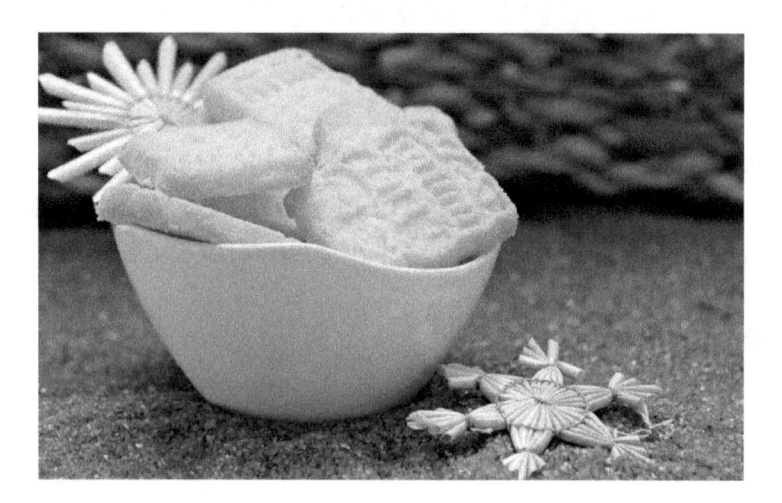

Give your regular coconut cookies a twist, add some grated pumpkin along with coconut, and enjoy your healthier cookie.

5. Pumpkin Masala Thepla

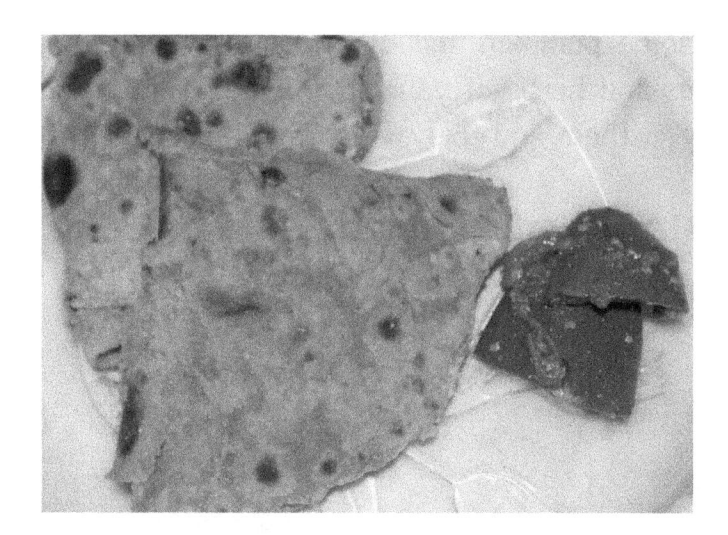

Add some grated pumpkin to your regular masala thepla, and enjoy this breakfast dish. (See the recipe section).

6. Whole-Grain Pumpkin Pancakes

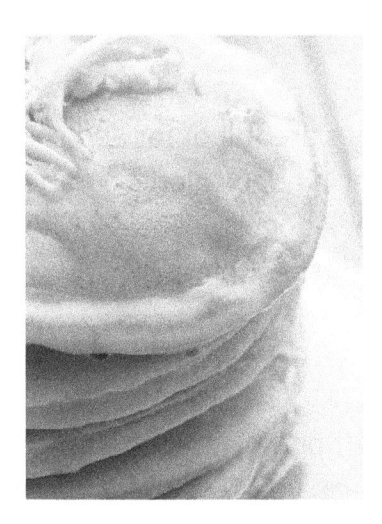

Perfect for winter, this hearty breakfast recipe includes whole-wheat flour, lots of spices, pumpkin, and milk.

7. Pumpkin Tikki

Grate some pumpkin and other veggies. Add some boiled potatoes and herbs of your choice. Roll it in breadcrumbs, shallow fry them, and enjoy with tomato sauce.

8. Pasta in Pumpkin Sauce

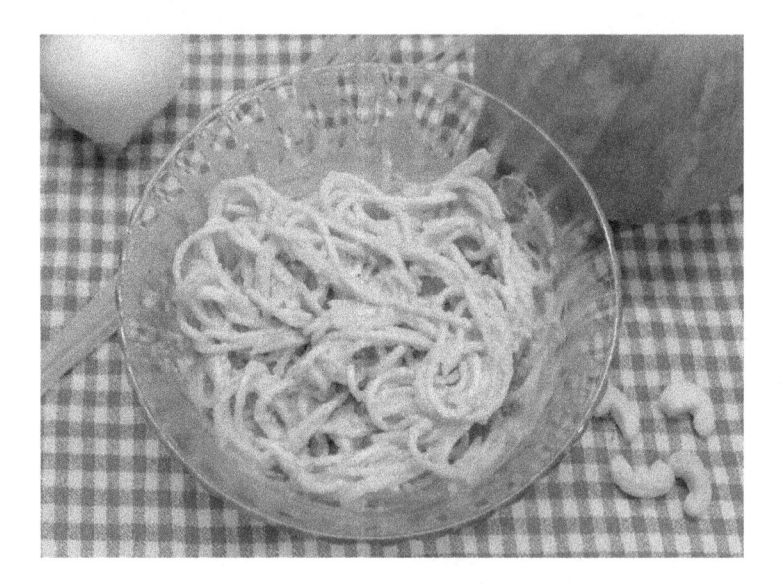

Creamy pasta dishes are full of fat and cholesterol. Instead of making your dinner a huge calorie bomb, try pumpkin cream sauce and use Greek yogurt instead of heavy cream to make your pasta tastier and healthier.

9. Pumpkin Almond Muffins

Start your day with pumpkin almond muffins. These mouth-watering muffins are a perfect snack on the go and will keep you in energy until it's time for lunch.

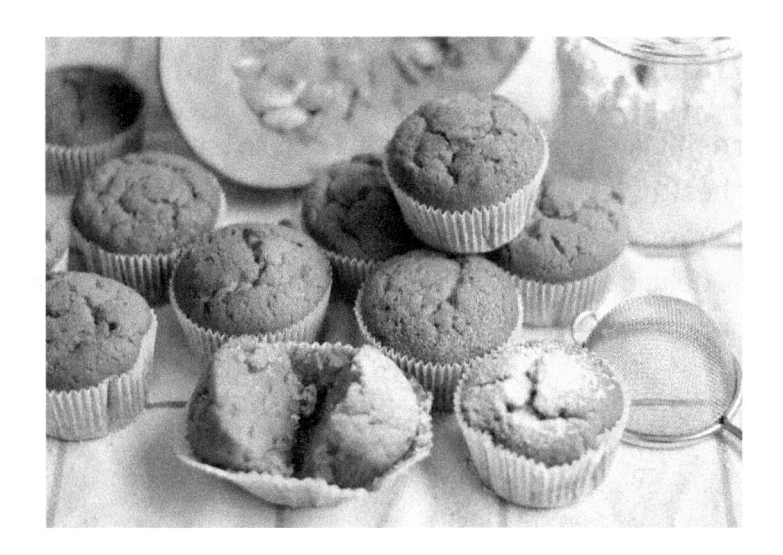

10. Pumpkin Waffles

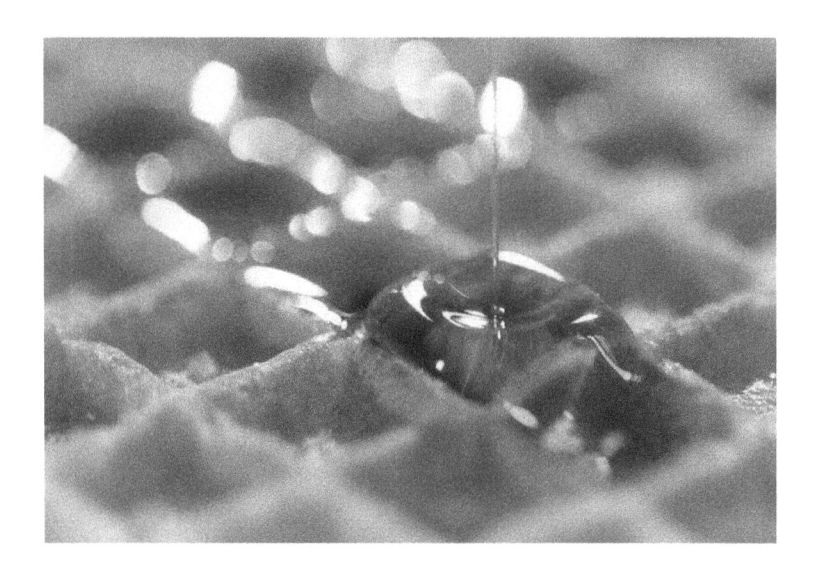

Combine all the dry ingredients: flour, sugar, baking soda, baking powder, and salt in a bowl and stir well. Add the wet ingredients: pumpkin, buttermilk, butter, vanilla essence, and mix until smooth. Preheat the waffle iron, brush it with melted butter, and cook waffles. Eat with toppings of your choice.

My Thoughts

If you don't like pumpkins but still want to eat them because of their health benefits, then these are my ideas of smartly incorporating pumpkins into the diet, which will be healthy as well as delicious. If you are already a pumpkin lover, here you got some more interesting recipes to add to your list.

CHAPTER 9

RECIPES

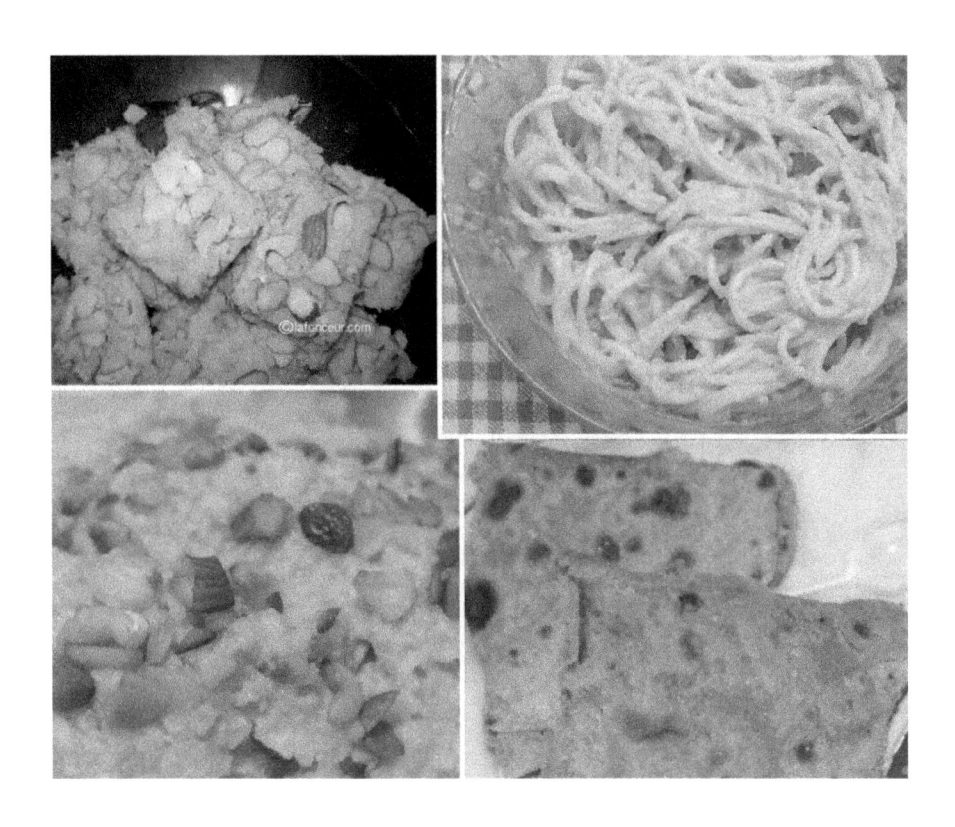

Coconut Burfi Sweet and Healthy

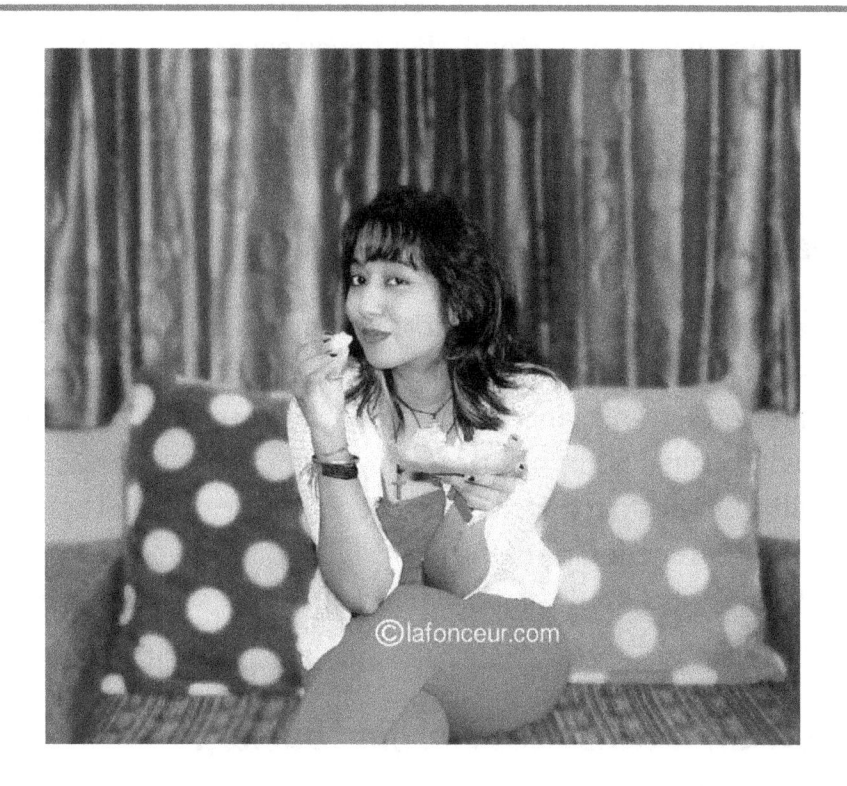

Coconut burfi is healthy because it has nuts. You can make it even healthier by substituting refined white sugar with brown sugar. If you use jaggery instead of brown sugar, it would be even more beneficial to your health. Also, replace normal unsalted butter with **ghee** (clarified butter made from cow's milk).

If you are health conscious but sweet tooth, coconut burfi is the best option you can go for without even second thought.

Health Benefits of Coconut Burfi:

Desiccated coconut:

We all know coconut contains fat but healthy fat, which is essential for body function. It lowers LDL levels (bad cholesterol) and increases good cholesterol or HDL, strengthening your arteries and promoting cardiovascular health. Other than that, it is very good for the skin and helps in the better functioning of the brain. It contains several essential nutrients, including dietary fiber, manganese, copper, and selenium.

Cow Ghee (Unsalted clarified butter):

As per Ayurved, cow Ghee is very good for health. Cow ghee is full of essential nutrients, healthy fats with antibacterial, antifungal, antioxidants, and antiviral properties. It normalizes Vata and Pitta and nourishes the body. It is known as a brain tonic. Excellent for improving memory power and intelligence. Ghee is best for strengthening mental health. It is beneficial for curing thyroid dysfunction. It heals wounds, chapped lips, and mouth ulcers and best for joints' lubrication. It cures insomnia.

But it should consume in moderation if you don't want to put on weight.

Jaggery:

Jaggery boosts immunity. The ability to purify the blood is the most well-known of all the benefits of jaggery. It is among the best natural cleansing agents for the body. It Prevents anemia, controls blood pressure, and prevents respiratory problems. Jaggery has a complex carbohydrate that gives energy to the body gradually and for a longer time, therefore, helps in preventing fatigue and weakness of the body.

How to make Coconut Burfi

Ingredients:
Desiccated coconut: 2 cups
Cow ghee (Unsalted clarified butter): 1 tablespoon
Cow's milk: 2 cups
Brown sugar/Jaggery: 3/4 cup
Saffron: a pinch
Shredded almonds: For decoration

Method:

Soak saffron in 2 tablespoons of hot milk. Keep aside. Dry roast desiccated coconut.

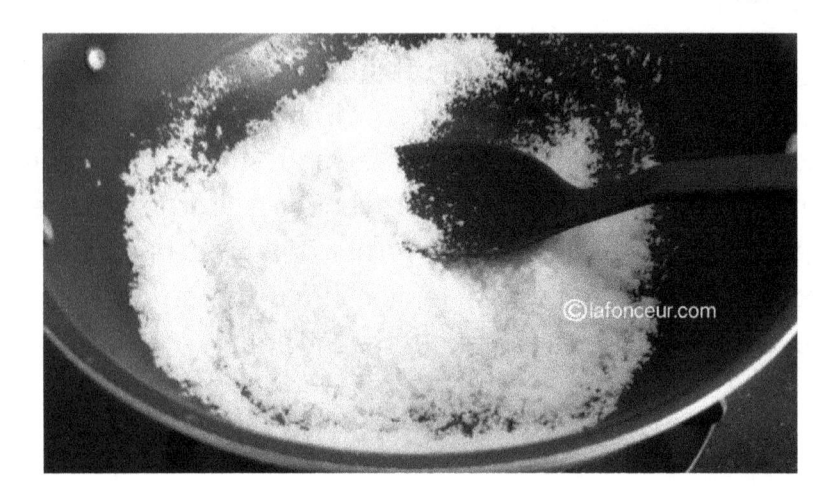

Heat 1 tablespoon Cow Ghee (Unsalted clarified butter).

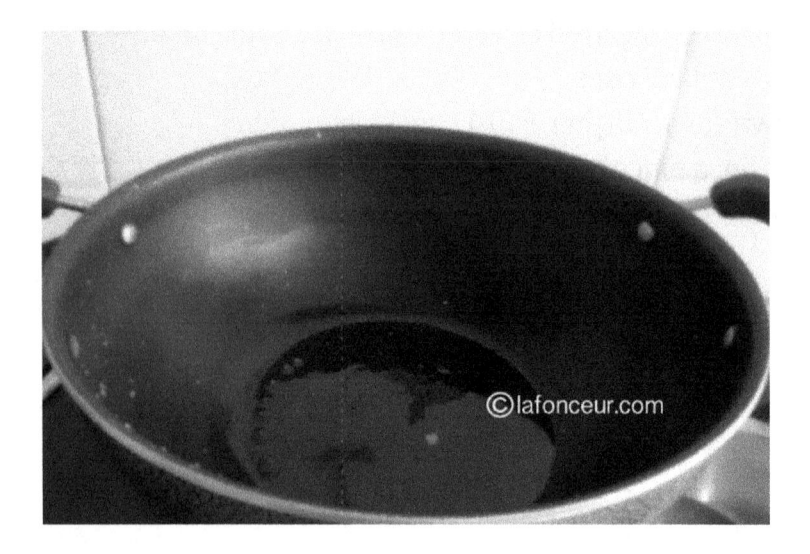

Add cow's milk.

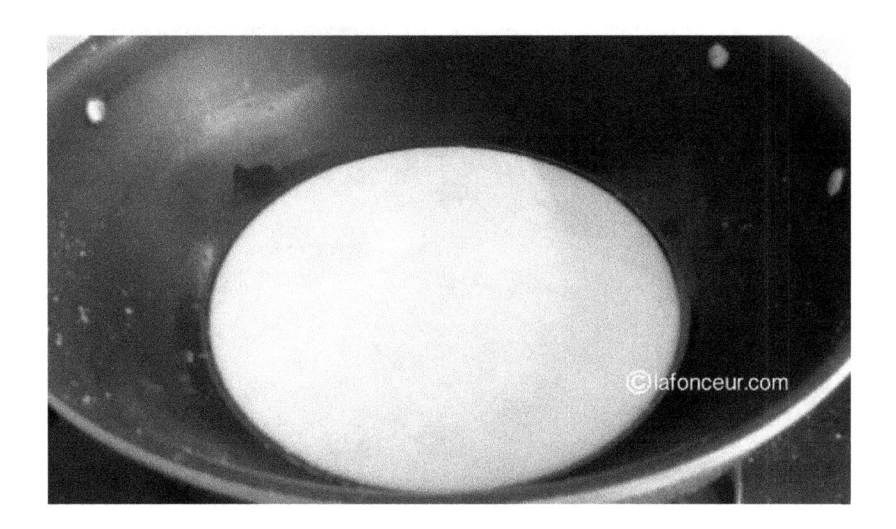

Bring it to a boil and reduce it to half.

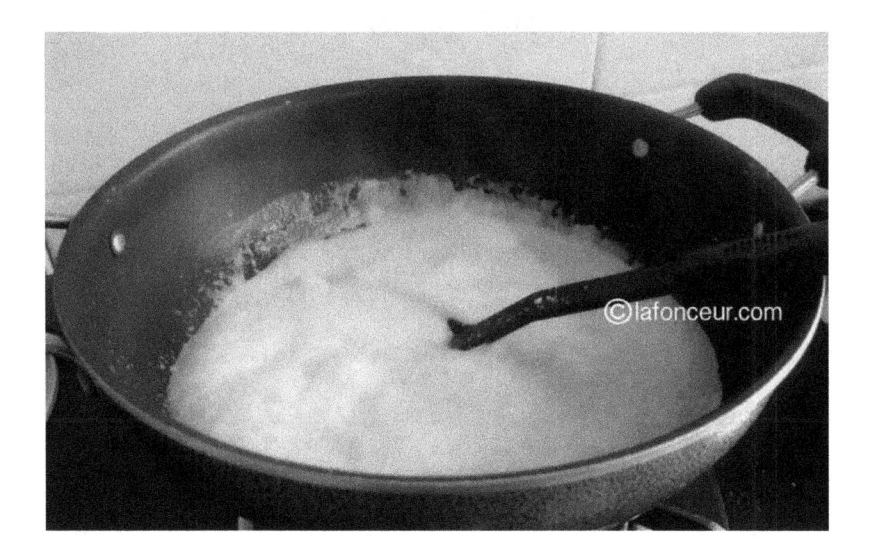

Add brown sugar or jaggery.

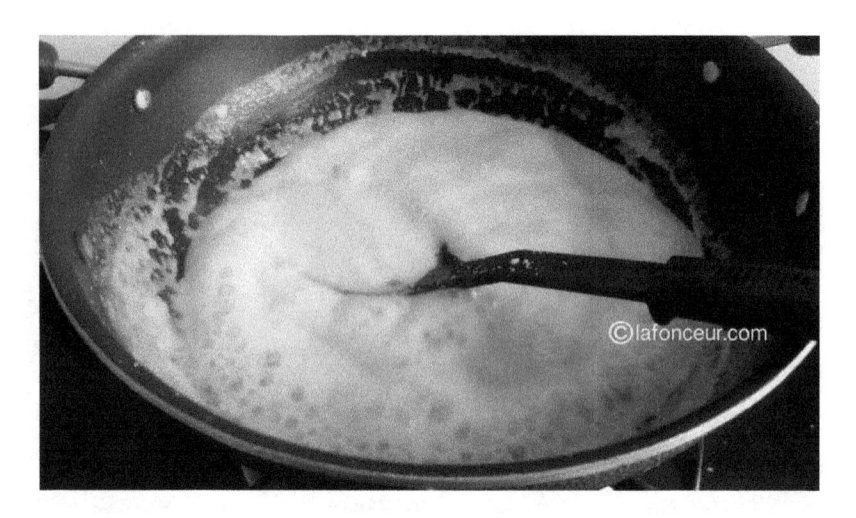

Add roasted desiccated coconut.

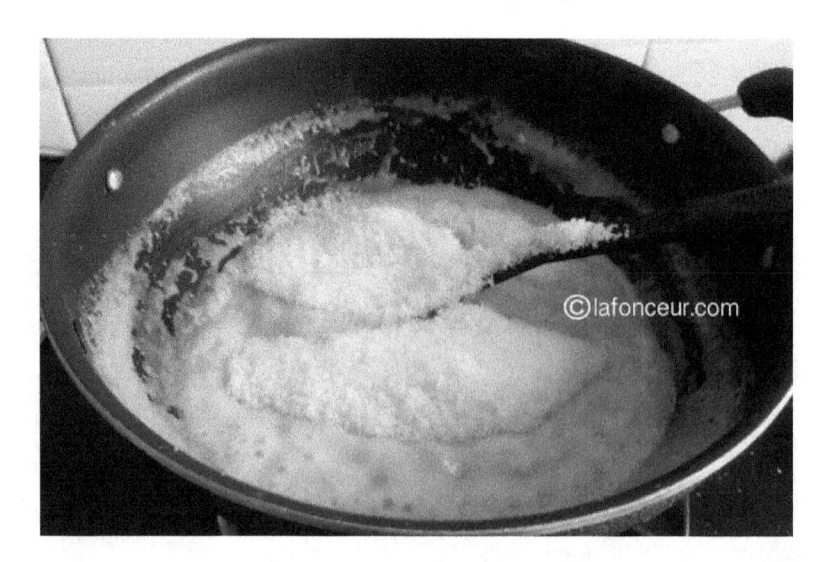

Mix well.

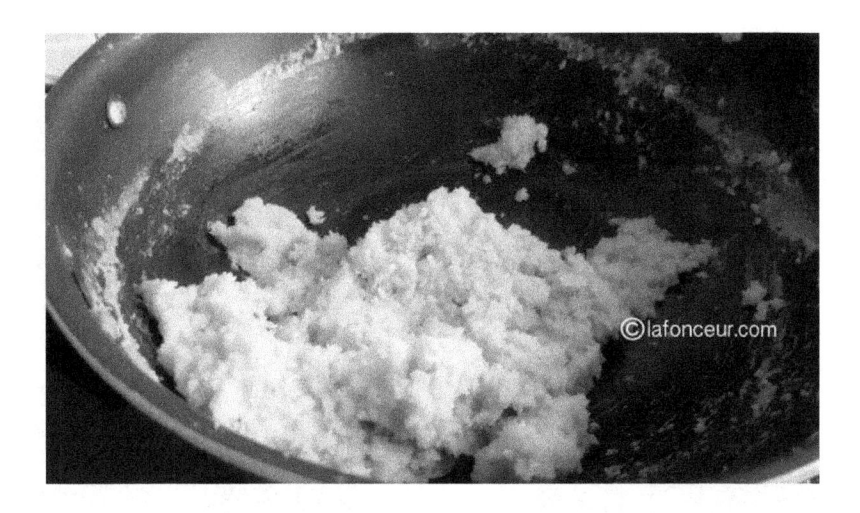

Add saffron soaked in milk.

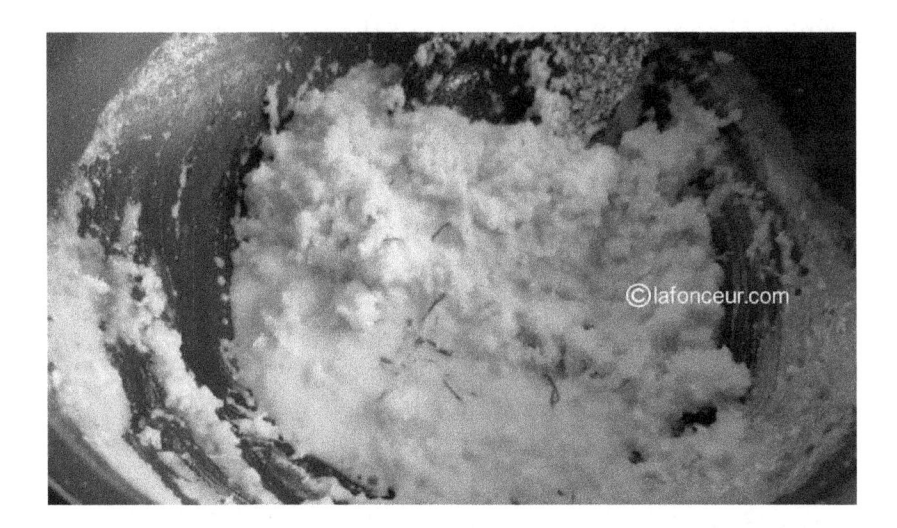

Pour it into a baking dish.

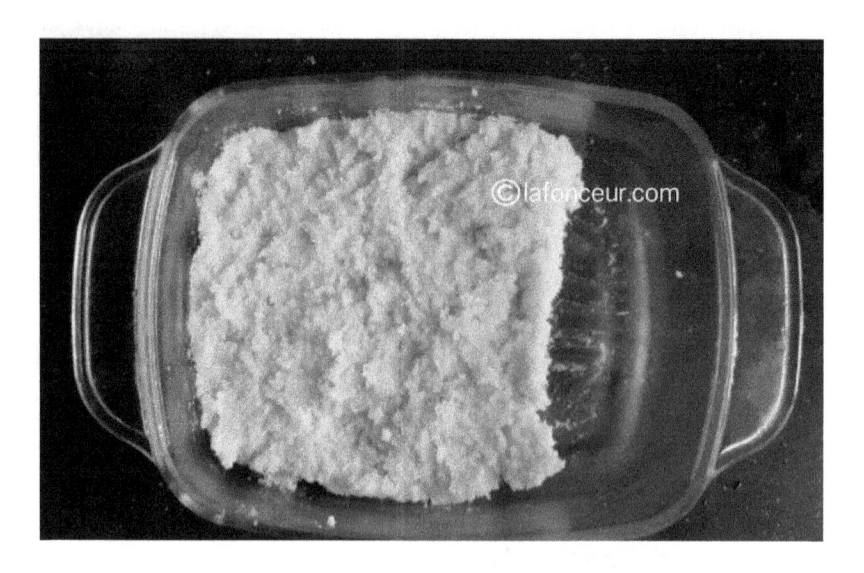

Sprinkle shredded almonds and cut them into squares.

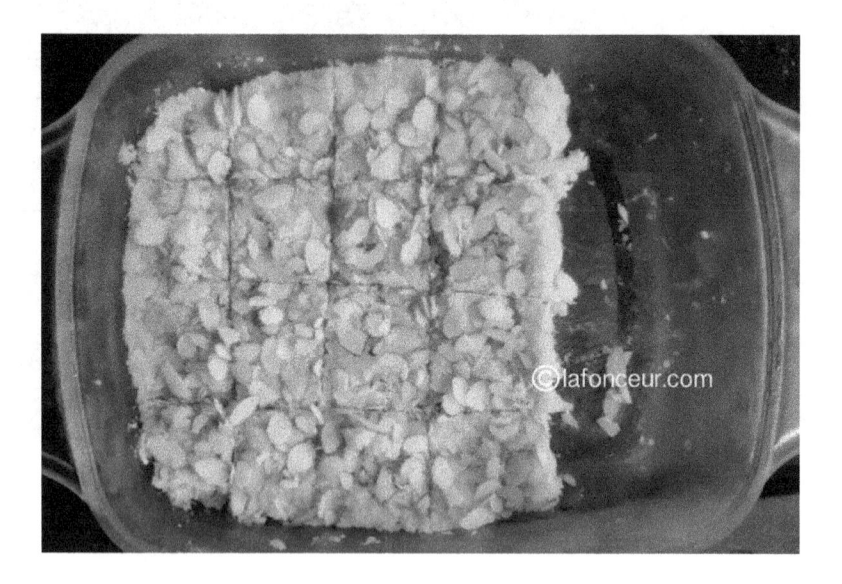

Refrigerate for 2 hours, and voila Coconut Burfi is ready to eat.

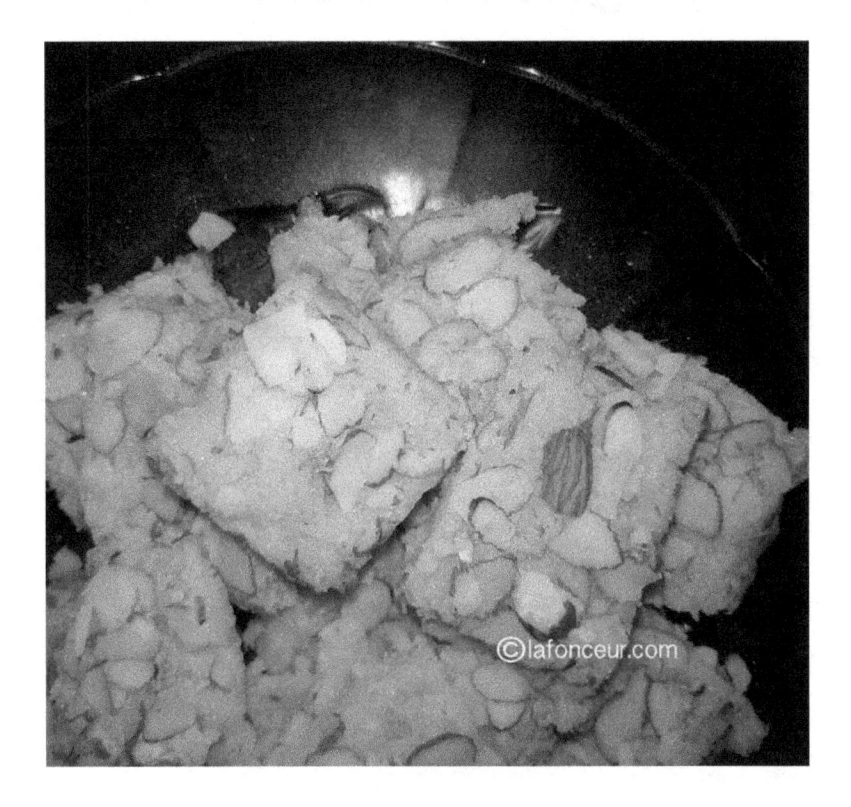

The best part of coconut burfi is you can consume it without worrying about your health. Do try yourself to satisfy your sweet craving.

Spaghetti in Creamy Pumpkin Sauce

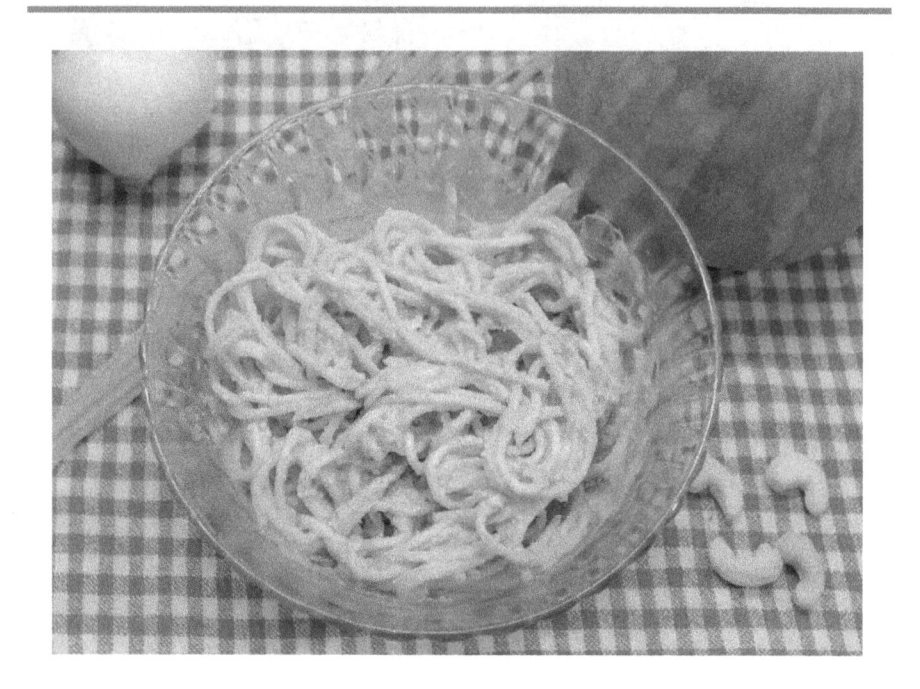

Serves: 2

Ingredients:

Cooked spaghetti: 200 gm

Pumpkin: 300 gm

Cashew nuts: ½ cup

Garlic: 5 cloves

White onion: 1 large

Red chili powder: ½ teaspoon

Black pepper: a pinch

Salt: To taste

Water: 1 cup

Olive oil: 2 tablespoons

Method:

For Pumpkin Puree

1. Take a pressure cooker. Add roughly chopped pumpkin and ½ cup water. Add salt. Pressure cook for 2 whistles.

2. Mash the pumpkin with a spatula.

For Pumpkin Sauce

1. Soak cashew nuts in ½ cup hot water for 15-20 mins. Drain the water and keep the soaked cashew nuts aside.

2. Take a pan. Add 2 tablespoons of olive oil. Heat it. Crush the garlic and immediately add it to the oil. Cook for 5 mins.

3. Add roughly chopped onion. Cook for 5-7 mins.

4. Add cashew nuts and cook for 3-5 mins.

5. Add pumpkin puree. Add red chili powder, black pepper, and salt (we have added salt in pumpkin puree too, so add accordingly).

6. Mix well. Cover the mixture with a lid and cook at low flame

for 10-15 mins. Mix in between so that the mixture doesn't stick to the bottom of the pan.

7. Turn off the flame and let the mix cool. Now blend until very smooth with ¼ cup of water. The sauce should be smooth, thick, and free from any lumps.

8. Take out the sauce in a bowl. Add cooked spaghetti and mix well. Your creamy and healthy spaghetti is ready to eat.

Note:

1. Crush garlic just before adding it to oil for enhanced garlic flavor.

2. Cook the pumpkin mix with the lid on for at least 10 mins to remove the raw taste of pumpkin and onion.

3. Use white onion because white onions are sweeter and milder than yellow onions and perfect for making sauce.

4. The smoother you blend the creamer will be your pumpkin sauce.

Pumpkin Halwa

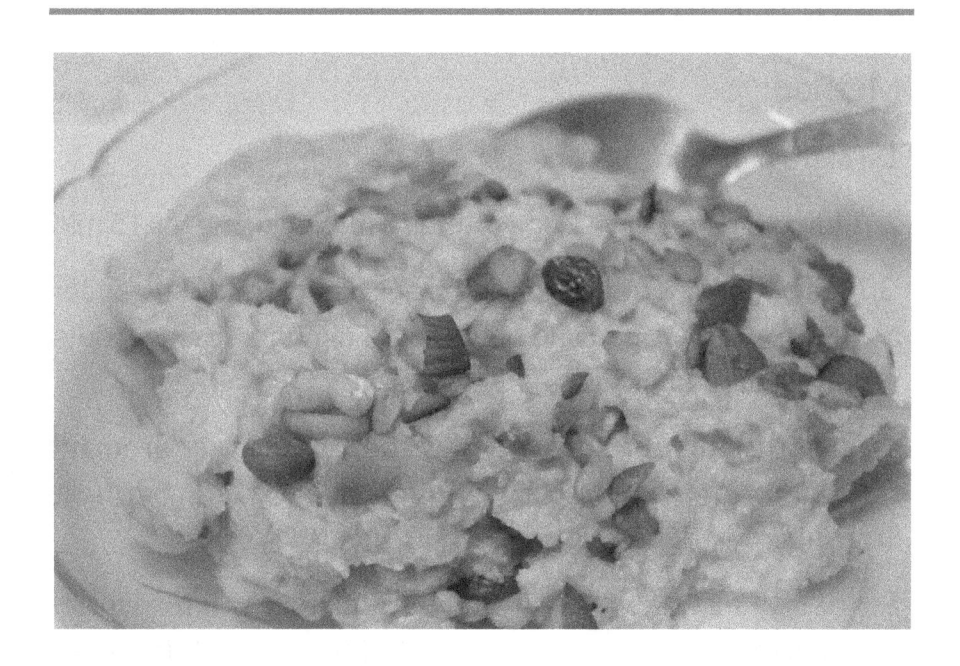

Ingredients:

Grated pumpkin: 500 gm

Milk: 500 ml

Almonds: 10-12

Cashew nuts: 10-12

Raisins 10-12

Melon seeds: 1 tablespoon

Jaggery: 100 gm or Brown sugar: ½ cup

Desiccated coconut: 3 tablespoons

Ghee: 1 teaspoon

Method:

1. Take a pan. Add milk and bring it to a boil.

2. Add grated pumpkin. Cook on medium-high flame for 15 min.

3. Meanwhile, chop almonds and cashew nuts. Take 1 teaspoon of ghee in another pan and heat it. Add almonds, cashew nuts, melon seeds, and raisins.

4. Sauté the nuts and seeds till they start releasing an aromatic smell and turn slightly brown. Remove the nuts from heat. Store in an air-tight container.

5. After 15 min the pumpkin and milk mixture will turn into a thick paste. Add jaggery and desiccated coconut at this stage.

6. Cook the halwa for another 10 min till it starts leaving the pan.

7. Turn off the flame. Let the pumpkin halwa cool. Refrigerate it for 2 hours. Sprinkle the nuts just before serving and enjoy this healthy and tasty dessert.

Pumpkin Masala Thepla

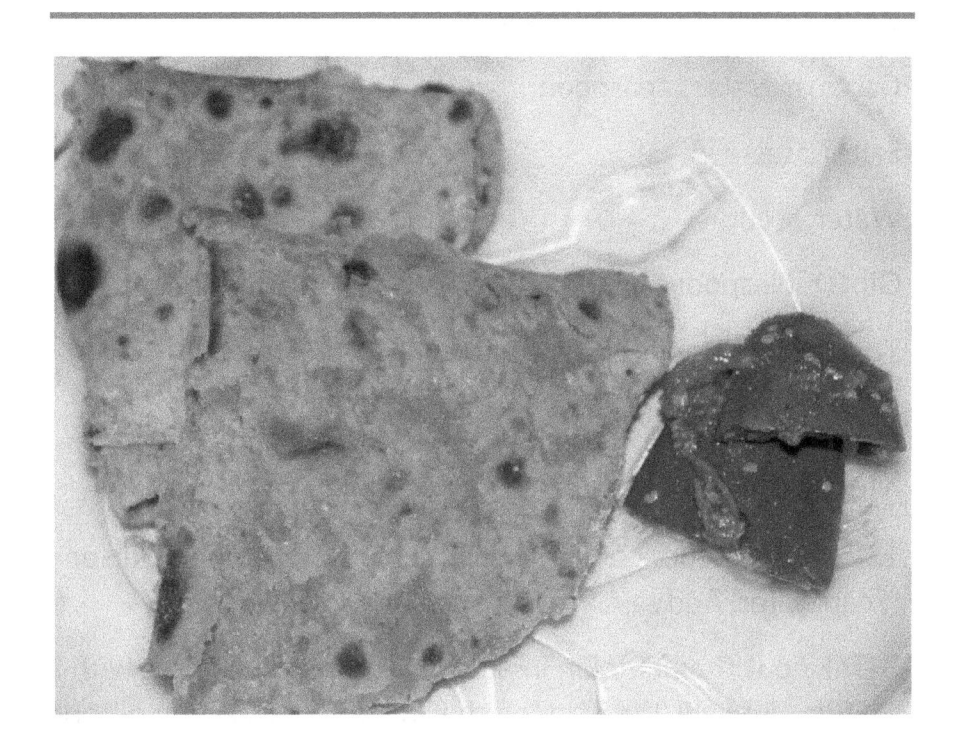

Serves: 2

Ingredients:

Pumpkin: 300 gm

Whole wheat flour: 1 cup

Millet flour: ½ cup

Chickpea flour: ½ cup

Turmeric powder: ½ teaspoon

Grated ginger: 1 tablespoon

Chopped green chilies: 1 teaspoon

White sesame seeds: 1 teaspoon

Garam masala: 1 teaspoon

Salt: To taste

Water: ½ cup

Oil: 3 tablespoons

Yogurt: 2 tablespoons (If required)

Method

1. Take a pressure cooker. Add roughly chopped pumpkin and ½ cup water. Add salt. Pressure cook for 2 whistles.

2. Take out the pumpkin in a bowl. Mash the pumpkin with a spatula. Add all the rest of the ingredients except oil and yogurt.

3. Knead to a soft dough. Pumpkin has high water content, plus we have added water while making the puree, so no additional water is required for kneading. But if your dough looks dry, add 1 to 2 tablespoons of thick yogurt.

4. Divide the dough into 8-9 equal parts. Make medium-sized dough balls.

5. Take one piece of the dough ball, dip it in the dry whole wheat flour, and dust off the excess flour.

6. Use a rolling pin to roll the dough into a thin 5 inches-6-inch circle.

7. Heat the pan/griddle (Tawa) on medium-high flame.

8. Place the thepla on the griddle. Cook for about a minute or cook until the thepla begins puffing up from the base at some places.

9. Flip the thepla and spread 3-4 drops of oil. Cook for 2 minutes until it turns light brown.

10. Flip the thepla again and top with 3-4 drops of oil, spreading it evenly over the surface. Gently press the thepla with the flat spatula to help it cook evenly.

11. Once brown spots are visible on both sides of the thepla, transfer it to a serving plate. Similarly, make all the theplas.

12. Enjoy pumpkin masala thepla with the pickle of your choice for breakfast.

ALSO READ

Eat So What! The Power of Vegetarianism

(The next book in the Eat So What! series)

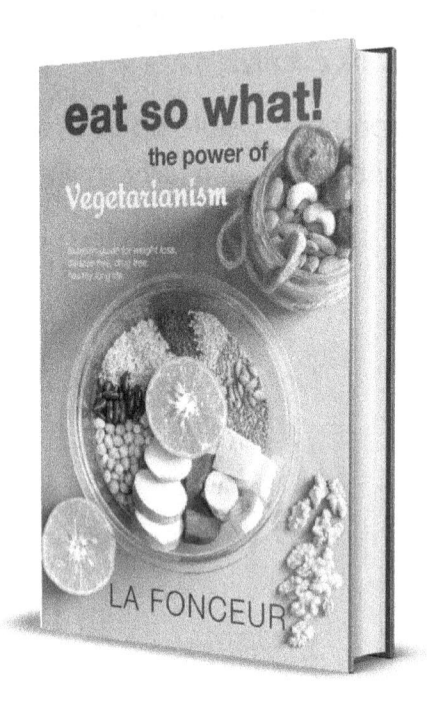

In Eat So What! The Power of Vegetarianism, understand your food scientifically and naturally overcome nutritional deficiencies without any dietary supplements!

NOTE FROM LA FONCEUR

Dear Reader,

Thank you for reading *Eat So What! Smart Ways to Stay Healthy*. I hope you have found this book helpful.

If you liked the book, please leave a short review online telling why you enjoyed reading it. This will help other health-conscious readers find this book. Your help in spreading awareness is gratefully received.

Join my mailing list at **www.eatsowhat.com/esw-mailing-list/** to receive offers and updates of my new release.

_____

Also, read how foods that work with the same mechanism as medicines can naturally prevent and control chronic diseases such as diabetes, hypertension and arthritis in *Eat to Prevent and Control Disease*.

If you are looking for a permanent solution to your hair problems, read *Secret of Healthy Hair*.

All of my books are available in eBook, paperback, and hardcover editions. Happy reading!

Regards

La Fonceur

ABOUT THE AUTHOR

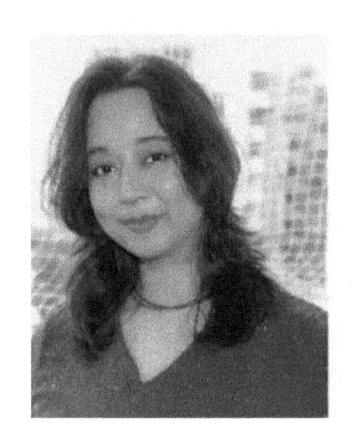

La Fonceur is the author of the book series *Eat So What!*, *Secret of Healthy Hair*, and *Eat to Prevent and Control Disease*. She is a health blogger and a dance artist. She has a master's degree in Pharmacy. She specialized in Pharmaceutical Technology and worked as a research scientist in the research and development department. She has published an article titled "Techniques for Producing Biotechnology-Derived Products of Pharmaceutical Use" in the Pharmtechmedica Journal. She is also a registered pharmacist. Being a research scientist, she has worked closely with drugs. Based on her experience, she believes that one can prevent most diseases with nutritious vegetarian foods and a healthy lifestyle.

ALL BOOKS BY LA FONCEUR

Full-length books:

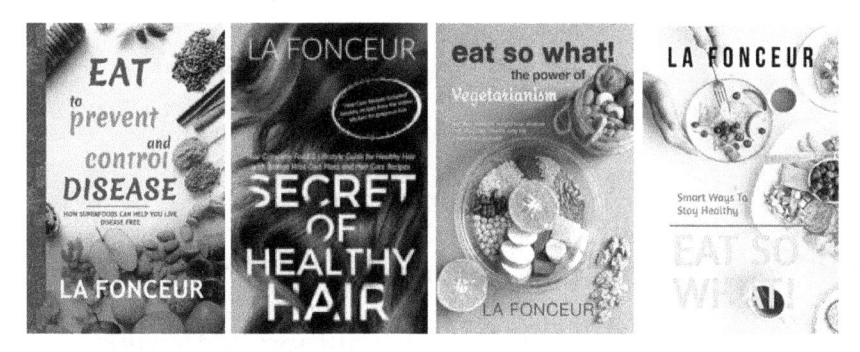

Mini extract editions:

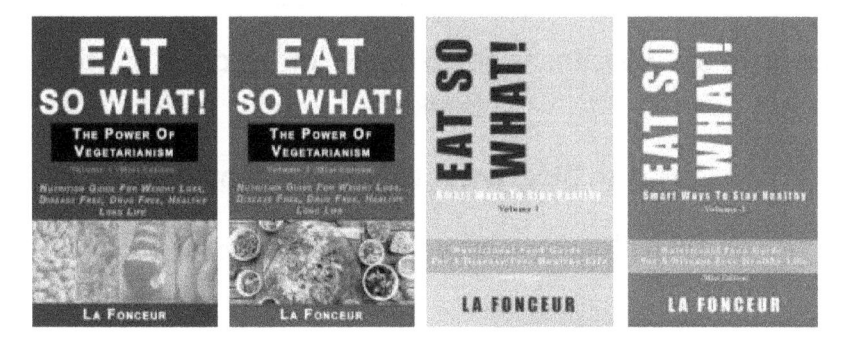

Hindi editions:

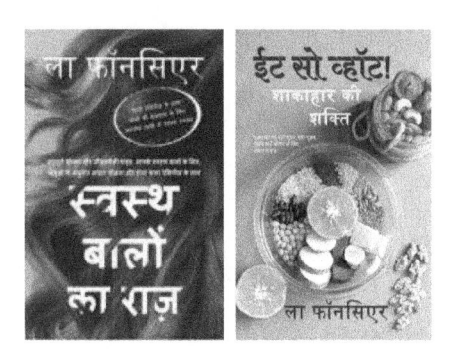

CONNECT WITH LA FONCEUR

Instagram: @la_fonceur | @eatsowhat

Facebook: **LaFonceur** | eatsowhat

Twitter: **@la_fonceur**

Amazon Author Page:

www.amazon.com/La-Fonceur/e/B07PM8SBSG/

Bookbub: www.bookbub.com/authors/la-fonceur

Sign up to the websites to get exclusive offers on La Fonceur eBooks:

Health Blog: www.eatsowhat.com

Website: www.lafonceur.com/sign-up

MONTHLY HEALTHY HABIT TRACKER

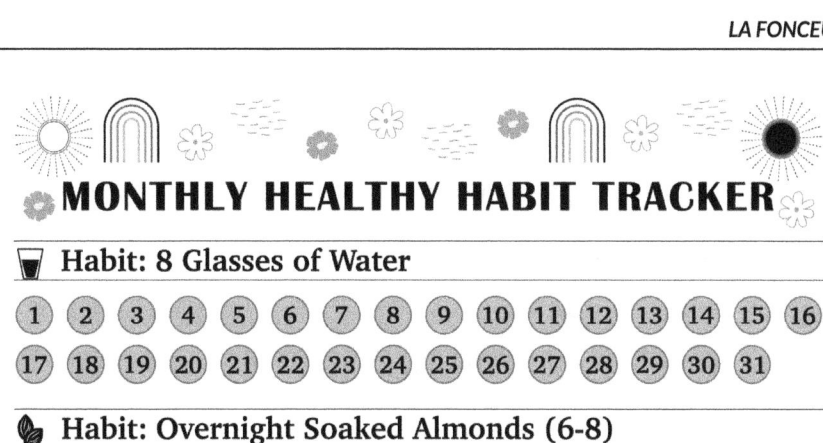

Habit: 8 Glasses of Water

① ② ③ ④ ⑤ ⑥ ⑦ ⑧ ⑨ ⑩ ⑪ ⑫ ⑬ ⑭ ⑮ ⑯
⑰ ⑱ ⑲ ⑳ ㉑ ㉒ ㉓ ㉔ ㉕ ㉖ ㉗ ㉘ ㉙ ㉚ ㉛

Habit: Overnight Soaked Almonds (6-8)

① ② ③ ④ ⑤ ⑥ ⑦ ⑧ ⑨ ⑩ ⑪ ⑫ ⑬ ⑭ ⑮ ⑯
⑰ ⑱ ⑲ ⑳ ㉑ ㉒ ㉓ ㉔ ㉕ ㉖ ㉗ ㉘ ㉙ ㉚ ㉛

Habit: 1-2 Fiber-Rich Foods

① ② ③ ④ ⑤ ⑥ ⑦ ⑧ ⑨ ⑩ ⑪ ⑫ ⑬ ⑭ ⑮ ⑯
⑰ ⑱ ⑲ ⑳ ㉑ ㉒ ㉓ ㉔ ㉕ ㉖ ㉗ ㉘ ㉙ ㉚ ㉛

Habit: 30 Minutes Walk

① ② ③ ④ ⑤ ⑥ ⑦ ⑧ ⑨ ⑩ ⑪ ⑫ ⑬ ⑭ ⑮ ⑯
⑰ ⑱ ⑲ ⑳ ㉑ ㉒ ㉓ ㉔ ㉕ ㉖ ㉗ ㉘ ㉙ ㉚ ㉛

Habit: 7-8 Hours of Sleep

① ② ③ ④ ⑤ ⑥ ⑦ ⑧ ⑨ ⑩ ⑪ ⑫ ⑬ ⑭ ⑮ ⑯
⑰ ⑱ ⑲ ⑳ ㉑ ㉒ ㉓ ㉔ ㉕ ㉖ ㉗ ㉘ ㉙ ㉚ ㉛

Habit:

① ② ③ ④ ⑤ ⑥ ⑦ ⑧ ⑨ ⑩ ⑪ ⑫ ⑬ ⑭ ⑮ ⑯
⑰ ⑱ ⑲ ⑳ ㉑ ㉒ ㉓ ㉔ ㉕ ㉖ ㉗ ㉘ ㉙ ㉚ ㉛

Habit:

① ② ③ ④ ⑤ ⑥ ⑦ ⑧ ⑨ ⑩ ⑪ ⑫ ⑬ ⑭ ⑮ ⑯
⑰ ⑱ ⑲ ⑳ ㉑ ㉒ ㉓ ㉔ ㉕ ㉖ ㉗ ㉘ ㉙ ㉚ ㉛

Habit:

① ② ③ ④ ⑤ ⑥ ⑦ ⑧ ⑨ ⑩ ⑪ ⑫ ⑬ ⑭ ⑮ ⑯
⑰ ⑱ ⑲ ⑳ ㉑ ㉒ ㉓ ㉔ ㉕ ㉖ ㉗ ㉘ ㉙ ㉚ ㉛

MONTHLY HEALTHY HABIT TRACKER

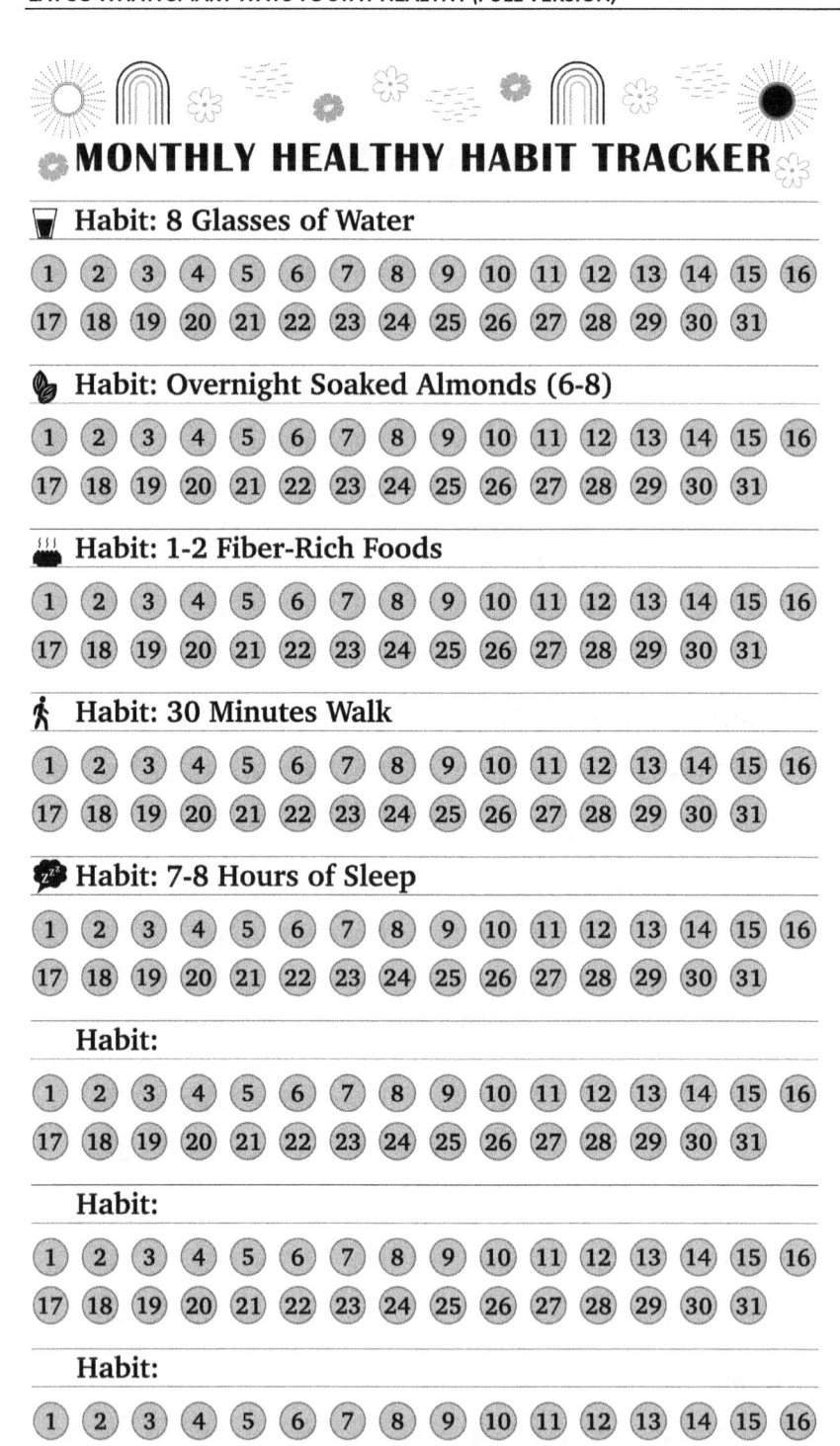

Habit: 8 Glasses of Water

① ② ③ ④ ⑤ ⑥ ⑦ ⑧ ⑨ ⑩ ⑪ ⑫ ⑬ ⑭ ⑮ ⑯
⑰ ⑱ ⑲ ⑳ ㉑ ㉒ ㉓ ㉔ ㉕ ㉖ ㉗ ㉘ ㉙ ㉚ ㉛

Habit: Overnight Soaked Almonds (6-8)

① ② ③ ④ ⑤ ⑥ ⑦ ⑧ ⑨ ⑩ ⑪ ⑫ ⑬ ⑭ ⑮ ⑯
⑰ ⑱ ⑲ ⑳ ㉑ ㉒ ㉓ ㉔ ㉕ ㉖ ㉗ ㉘ ㉙ ㉚ ㉛

Habit: 1-2 Fiber-Rich Foods

① ② ③ ④ ⑤ ⑥ ⑦ ⑧ ⑨ ⑩ ⑪ ⑫ ⑬ ⑭ ⑮ ⑯
⑰ ⑱ ⑲ ⑳ ㉑ ㉒ ㉓ ㉔ ㉕ ㉖ ㉗ ㉘ ㉙ ㉚ ㉛

Habit: 30 Minutes Walk

① ② ③ ④ ⑤ ⑥ ⑦ ⑧ ⑨ ⑩ ⑪ ⑫ ⑬ ⑭ ⑮ ⑯
⑰ ⑱ ⑲ ⑳ ㉑ ㉒ ㉓ ㉔ ㉕ ㉖ ㉗ ㉘ ㉙ ㉚ ㉛

Habit: 7-8 Hours of Sleep

① ② ③ ④ ⑤ ⑥ ⑦ ⑧ ⑨ ⑩ ⑪ ⑫ ⑬ ⑭ ⑮ ⑯
⑰ ⑱ ⑲ ⑳ ㉑ ㉒ ㉓ ㉔ ㉕ ㉖ ㉗ ㉘ ㉙ ㉚ ㉛

Habit:

① ② ③ ④ ⑤ ⑥ ⑦ ⑧ ⑨ ⑩ ⑪ ⑫ ⑬ ⑭ ⑮ ⑯
⑰ ⑱ ⑲ ⑳ ㉑ ㉒ ㉓ ㉔ ㉕ ㉖ ㉗ ㉘ ㉙ ㉚ ㉛

Habit:

① ② ③ ④ ⑤ ⑥ ⑦ ⑧ ⑨ ⑩ ⑪ ⑫ ⑬ ⑭ ⑮ ⑯
⑰ ⑱ ⑲ ⑳ ㉑ ㉒ ㉓ ㉔ ㉕ ㉖ ㉗ ㉘ ㉙ ㉚ ㉛

Habit:

① ② ③ ④ ⑤ ⑥ ⑦ ⑧ ⑨ ⑩ ⑪ ⑫ ⑬ ⑭ ⑮ ⑯
⑰ ⑱ ⑲ ⑳ ㉑ ㉒ ㉓ ㉔ ㉕ ㉖ ㉗ ㉘ ㉙ ㉚ ㉛

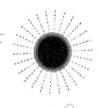

NOTES

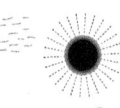

NOTES

Lightning Source UK Ltd.
Milton Keynes UK
UKHW020010091122
411848UK00014B/594